Walsh was able to see the beauty in life.
He spent his valuable time helping us to open our eyes'

Cecelia Ahern

Fionnbar Walsh is married to Elma Walsh and father of Jema and Donal. He lives in County Kerry.

DONAL'S MOUNTAIN

Fionnbar Walsh

sphere

SPHERE

First published in Great Britain in 2014 by Sphere

Written with June Considine

Lyrics from 'Home from the Sea' used with permission
of Phil Coulter/Four Seasons Music Ltd

Excerpt from 'The Road Not Taken' by Robert Frost used
with permission of Henry Holt and Company, New York

A CIP catalogue record for this book
is available from the British Library.

ISBN 978-0-7515-5679-7

Typeset in Cambria and Calibri by Bookends Publishing Ltd
Printed and bound in Great Britain by
Clays Ltd, St Ives Plc

Papers used by Sphere are from well-managed forests
and other responsible sources.

MIX
Paper from
responsible sources
FSC
www.fsc.org   FSC® C104740

Sphere
An imprint of
Little, Brown Book Group
100 Victoria Embankment
London EC4Y 0DY

An Hachette UK Company
www.hachette.co.uk

www.littlebrown.co.uk

Contents

To Elma and Jema,
my rock and crutches on this journey!

Author's Note

My son Donal wrote a school essay about his battle with cancer that was published in the CBS The Green Yearbook and later appeared in a local newspaper, the *Kerry's Eye*, along with his appeal to young people to value life. Following his appearance on *The Saturday Night Show*, he was asked by the *Sunday Independent* to update his essay. This was published in the *Sunday Independent* under the headline 'My Struggle with Cancer', along with his essay, 'Climbing God's Mountain', and the 'suicide letter' (an appeal to young people to value life) that he wrote shortly before his death. Donal's writings have been incorporated into this book.

Prologue

I've climbed God's mountains, faced many struggles for my life and dealt with so much loss. And as much as I'd love to go around to every fool on this planet and open their eyes to the mountains that surround them in life, I can't. But maybe if I shout from mine, they'll pay attention.

Donal Walsh, 1996–2013

'Why me?' Donal asked. 'Why does it have to be me?'

Cancer, 'the big C', the dreaded word, and our twelve-year-old son was asking us, his parents, a question we found impossible to answer.

'Why me?'

That same question asked, again and again. All we could do was hug him, hold and support him, and reassure him that we would get through this ordeal together. We did our weeping in private and in the midst of our bewilderment, we looked at each other and asked, 'Why us?'

This is a story about an invasion into our lives. The story of our son, Donal Walsh, who took on a battle of heroic proportions and who, over the four years that followed his asking us that first unanswerable question, was able to say, 'If this is what God wants me to do – if he wants me to fight cancer, if he wants me to be a symbol to other people or if he just wants me to die – then I guess I'll strap up my hiking boots and get to the top of this mountain.'

In the final months before his death, our son spoke frankly in a television interview about his cancer and how he had accepted the terminal prognosis. He also expressed the anger he felt over the loss of young lives through suicide. His own life would be taken from him before he reached his seventeenth birthday. He had no choice in the matter, and it grieved him that young people who were going through troubled times could not see any value in their own lives. He pleaded with them to find a door in their darkness and to reach out for help. Their lives were too precious to be squandered, he believed, and it was this appeal, along with the courage he displayed when speaking about his own impending death, that created such an immediate impact. In this age of instant online communication, this simple yet thoughtful message – that suicide is a permanent solution to a temporary problem – instigated a conversation that spread like wildfire on Facebook and Twitter and other media outlets. That conversation is still continuing today, but our son is no longer here to engage with it. Shortly after that interview, he lost his fight for life. He left behind an abiding memory of his bravery as he faced into the most difficult journey of his young life.

In the poem, 'The Road Not Taken' by Robert Frost, the poet wrote:

I shall be telling this with a sigh
Somewhere ages and ages hence:
Two roads diverged in a wood, and I —
I took the one less travelled by,
And that has made all the difference.

Two roads diverged for Donal. He took the one less travelled by – and walked valiantly along its course until he reached the end of his journey and was carried into the light.

I tell you his story with a sigh, but also with tremendous pride. It is my tribute to my son, who became a man as he journeyed along his road less travelled.

Fionnbar Walsh

PART ONE
KNOWING DONAL

Chapter One

The atmosphere in Dublin's Four Seasons Hotel is expectant and celebratory. It's early November 2013 and the media have gathered together on this afternoon to acknowledge the outstanding work done by their colleagues throughout the year. The National Newspapers of Ireland Awards ceremony is an annual highlight in the media calendar, and this is the first time my wife Elma and I have been invited to attend the event.

We recognise many of the faces surrounding us. We've seen them on television, heard their voices on radio, we've seen their bylines in print. Familiar names are announced and those in question rise to receive their awards: Kitty Holland, Fintan O'Toole, Paul Williams, Fionnan Sheahan, Tom Lyons and others, who are here today to be rewarded for their exceptional contributions to journalism. We've read their stories and discussed the issues they raised, and now we join in with the applause that greets each announcement.

Soon it is our turn. Some months ago we would have been nervous at such a formal occasion. But since Donal's death, we've been invited to a number of such events and we've become accustomed to cameras flashing, to the applause and the long walk between the tables to the stage. Brendan O'Connor, the journalist and television chat show host, presents us with the award, which we are accepting on behalf of our son. Brendan is a familiar face by now and he, more than anyone else at this gala celebration, has a deep awareness of exactly what this award means to us. It was on *The Saturday Night Show* that our son, Donal Walsh, first shot to national prominence and that occasion changed our lives in ways we could not have envisaged.

Brendan, on behalf of the awards committee, speaks eloquently and movingly about Donal. 'Some people live all their lives without ever acquiring a real sense of what they are about,' he says. 'Donal Walsh lived among us a mere sixteen years and, by the time of his parting, had bequeathed us a wisdom to serve the ages.'

Sometimes, on occasions such as this, we find it difficult to recognise the son we knew and loved. He sounds saintly and wise beyond his years, yet to us he was an ordinary boy, romping through life until fate decreed another direction for him.

As Brendan continues the speech, I try to hold back my tears. I think of Donal and how thrilled he would be if he, instead of us, was standing here to receive this award. To have his writing recognised by his peers – nothing would have pleased him more. When his articles were published in the *Sunday Independent*, he photographed the pages, so that he could carry them with him everywhere, on his mobile phone. He whooped with delight when he was paid for this work. But this is a posthumous award and, as such, the silence of the audience is weighted with respect and sympathy for our loss.

'To an Ireland down-at-heel materially and spiritually, Donal Walsh's words were a reminder to us to count our blessings and be thankful for the simple things in life,' says Brendan, as he hands the award to Elma. 'Donal, the Celestial Tiger, will forever burn bright in our memory for teaching us to value what we have – when we have it. That is why Donal Walsh has won the Outstanding Contribution to Public Debate award.'

The applause which follows resonates with compassion for us, but also with an enthusiastic appreciation for what Donal managed to achieve in his short life. The cameras begin to flash once more, as we pose for photographs, smile and shake hands.

When the ceremonial part of the afternoon ends, people offer us their congratulations, their condolences and, in some instances, their stories. Again, this is something with which we have become familiar: others sharing their experiences with us. Donal's openness struck such a chord with people that they feel easy speaking to us about their own, or their loved ones', darkest hours – and the courage needed to be able to shine a light into those shadows.

The afternoon has been a tremendous success. Some journalists are probably disappointed that their stories did not merit an award – but there is always next year, always another story.

When Donal died six months ago, we believed that his story was over. But since his passing, it has continued, in ways we could never have imagined. This is the reason we are here in this plush hotel where, for a short time, we can forget that our hearts have been shattered. We can forget that all we want – *really* want – is to wind the clock back. To be at home in Kerry within our familiar walls, listening to the sounds that knit a home together. We want to hear our son and daughter laughing, arguing, making up, sharing the gossip of the day. We want to hear the stereo playing too loudly from Donal's room, the beat of his drums from the shed, the clatter of his footsteps on the stairs, his cheers as Munster score a try, his groans when he is forced to sit still and finish his homework.

But we know that this is not possible, and so we smile and mingle and proudly hold out our son's award for people to admire. This is our new normality. What forces are directing us? Is it Donal's spirit at our shoulders or the power of his words that, once uttered, created a new energy that has entrusted us with the responsibility of keeping his legacy alive?

The outcome of even our most carefully planned decisions is in the hands of fate and we cannot predict the path our lives will take. Over twenty years ago I shaped my own future, when I decided to settle in Kerry. I was introduced to a community who would carry me and my beloved family through the very best of times and the darkest of days. The soul of this community never wavered in its support when the heartache came. A heartache which was the stuff of every parent's worst imaginings – a heartache we could never have anticipated.

Chapter Two

'You won't get out of Kerry without a ring on your finger,' my friends warned me when they heard I was moving to 'The Kingdom' to work in the hotel industry. Those were prophetic words, and no one seemed surprised when I met my wife Elma in 1991. We met at work – in the Brandon Hotel, where Elma worked in the accounts office. She was on holidays in the United States when I first arrived to take up my new position as Conference and Banqueting Manager at the hotel. We were introduced to each other when she returned to work and, not too long after that first meeting, I asked her out. She was late for our first date by a week and an hour! I'd like to pretend she was caught up in a serious emergency but the truth is … she *forgot*. This was not an auspicious beginning to our relationship but I persisted, and by the time she eventually turned up, I was hooked.

Elma was brought up on a farm outside Tralee, in a townland called The Kerries. I came from Knocklong in County Limerick, where I was one of six sons and a daughter. Elma was the only girl in a family of five brothers, so both of us thrived in the rough and tumble of a largely masculine environment. I played rugby, football and hurling throughout my childhood, and continued playing rugby until I was twenty-six. I loved the intensity of the scrum, the drive of the maul, the frenzy of the ruck. When I spent some time in Italy, I played internationally with the Rome Exiles. I'm still a passionate follower of the Munster rugby team and my heart swells with pride whenever I hear the roar from Thomond Park, where, as far as I'm concerned, all the great matches are and have been played.

I settled quickly into the Kerry lifestyle, which is an easy thing to do, as any 'blow-in' – and there are many – will testify. Elma, having finally decided to turn up for our first date, accepted my proposal of marriage two years after we started going out together. She did not have to decide whether or not she would take my surname, as her maiden name was also Walsh. And so when we exchanged our wedding vows, she remained Elma Walsh.

Our first year of married life was hectic, by any stretch of the imagination. I now had a new job and was responsible for supervising the construction of a new hotel. We were also ambitious enough to want to build our own house at the same time. Each project had its share of stresses and snag lists but, in the midst of all this activity, we still found time to enjoy our first baby – our spirited and adorable daughter, Jema.

Looking back on that first year, I wonder how we managed to cope, especially when, twenty-three months after Jema's arrival, along came Donal. How can I describe him? Feisty and full of energy, competitive, always hungry, loveable and determined to walk before he could crawl. At six weeks of age, he was eating solid food and had expressed a definite preference for potatoes. Fuel for his formidable energy, I guess. He was a complete contrast to Jema, who was a much calmer child and very tolerant of this boisterous younger brother, who had not only dethroned her from her position as the only child but seemed determined to compete with her at every level. The twenty-three-month age gap between them meant nothing to him. He was frustrated because she could talk and communicate with us, while he could not; frustrated that she could run around, while he was forced to crawl. And this meant he was on his feet and running by the time he was ten months old.

The new millennium was just beginning when we moved from our first home in Ballyrickard in Tralee to Blennerville, where we still live today. Blennerville is famous for its distinctive white windmill, the tallest of its kind in Europe. The view from our front window overlooks the Tralee Ship Canal that once ferried passengers and freight across Tralee Bay to the town. The canal fell into disuse for many years but has now been restored. Today it is mainly used by the Tralee Rowing Club, and the towpath is a popular place for dog-walkers and joggers. Beyond that, we can see the distant peaks of the Slieve Mish Mountains rising above the Atlantic. This view changes with the weather – awesomely beautiful on a clear day, or drenched in mist when the clouds swoop down, as they do with startling regularity, only to disappear just as swiftly. This view inspired Donal in many ways – but more about that later.

When we moved to Blennerville, Donal was four years old and delighted to be living so close to Elma's parents, Sheila and Mossie, and her brother Brendan. The family farm became a second home to Jema and Donal and their ever-growing band of cousins, some of them local, others from Dublin and Wicklow but who were regular visitors in the summer. The farmhouse was the heart of the family. This was where everyone gathered, sometimes to eat Sunday dinner or simply to get together for a chat while the cousins ran wild together through the fields, playing games of hide-and-seek behind barns and bales of hay. Mossie taught them to play cards and Sheila was the one who listened to their stories. If any of the kids had a fall, she would bandage their knees and pop a peppermint into their mouths to stop their tears. The nearby farm, belonging to Brian, Brendan's twin brother, was another favourite place to hang out and Brian developed a close, lasting relationship with both Donal and Jema.

Both of our children attended Spa National School. At four years of age, Donal was the second youngest in his class; however, as he was also one of the tallest, he was often mistaken for being older. I guess he was a 'teacher's pet'. His teachers loved him and he loved them in return. His primary school years were happy ones. I never heard him complain about having to go to school, and he went off happily in the mornings with his schoolbag on his back. He was a bright child, eager to learn. He soaked up information and retained it, which proved particularly helpful some years later, when he and three other pupils reached the finals in the All-Ireland Credit Union Schools Quiz.

After Donal started school, Elma decided to return to work with the accountancy firm Casey & Co. Accountants in Tralee. This company would later prove to be an invaluable source of understanding and support for us when the bleak times came. But in those early days, we had no idea of the shadows that would later form on our horizon. Jema and Donal were thriving in the freedom of rural life and the discipline of the sports field.

The passion of Kerry people for football needs no elaboration. Elma is an avid supporter of the Kerry team and our children were soon involved in the local Gaelic Athletic Association. Donal was four years old when he started playing Gaelic football for Kerins O'Rahillys GAA club, nicknamed the 'Naries', and volunteer-led, like all GAA clubs around Ireland. Donal and Jema were soon involved in many of the club's sporting activities. They played competitively from an early age and, over the following years, became County and Town Champions at junior level. One of Donal's proudest sporting achievements was winning a medal in the Under-12 GAA County Championship.

But, being a Limerick man, rugby was in my blood of course, and I was anxious to introduce Donal to the game at the earliest opportunity. He joined the Tralee Rugby Football Club when he was also four years old. As with everything else in his life, he took to the game immediately, with great energy. I'd some experience in coaching underage teams, so I was soon involved in training the younger players there. The club has prospered over the years and is now one of the largest and most successful in Munster, with about 500 children turning up each week for training.

I decided at an early stage however that it would be better for Donal if he was not in my squad. He knew how to twist me around his little finger, and I knew he'd play up any knocks or bruises he received. I also knew that, if my son was looking pleadingly at me from the ranks of hopefuls, it would be hard to be objective when choosing the best team to face the opposition.

Donal was quite happy to be trained by another coach. This gave him freedom from my watchful eye, but I monitored his progress closely and was delighted to see him developing his natural talent. I had a glimpse of the young man he would become on one occasion when a fight broke out during a match with a Limerick team. Surprisingly enough, the fight was not between the opposing sides, but took place among the Limerick players when they began to lose the match. Donal decided to intercede and talk his opponents back to the game. He seemed oblivious to the blows being exchanged and only reluctantly gave up his peace-making efforts when I intervened and ordered him back to his own side, and safety.

His height and strength made him a natural for a second-row forward. He played in the number 4 or 5 position, and was skilled at leaping for the ball in the line-out. We loved talking about rugby and attending matches together, especially at Thomond Park when Donal was older. On the way home he would sing with great gusto, and it could be anything from the latest rapper's rhymes to a ballad by Johnny Cash or Luke Kelly and The Dubliners. He watched videos of rugby matches and studied the techniques of his favourite players – like Paul O'Connell, who is recognised as one of the best second rows in world rugby. Donal also watched the All Blacks matches – they were probably his favourite team after Munster – and he was inspired by their discipline.

It seemed that nothing could stand in Donal's way or slow him down. Elma and I enjoyed being on the sidelines, cheering our children on at whatever game they were playing, and one, if not both of us, always accompanied them to their matches. Jema, who was equally keen on sport, won two County League medals and was picked for her school basketball team. Unfortunately, due to an injury, she was unable to continue playing competitively but her interest in sport is undiminished.

Unlike Donal, who was unable to stay still, Jema enjoys reading and spending quiet times by herself. His only nod to literature was a fascination with the Harry Potter books. He read the entire series and was as anxious as every young person in the country for the next book to come out. He enjoyed reading the occasional sports biography, but getting through them was a slow and sometimes torturous process. He much preferred to be up and about, and always doing something physical. Even attending the cinema constrained him, unless he was really interested in the film.

Time flew by, or so it seemed, as we celebrated another Christmas, another birthday, another year. My job changed a number of times but I stayed in the hospitality industry. Sometimes I had to work away from home for long stretches but, on the positive side, I was able to spend more time with my family in the tourist off-season. Our children never wanted for anything but we did not automatically buy them the latest toy or gadget. If they desired something badly enough, we encouraged them to save for it and they appreciated it all the more when they finally had it in their hands. We'd computers in the house for work purposes and both Jema and Donal were computer literate from an early age. I suppose you could call it an idyllic childhood, with many happy times and just the occasional low point, which never lasted long. Our mortgage was paid and our children were flourishing in a secure, loving environment.

The first shadow came with the deaths of Sheila and Mossie. Donal was nine years old when they fell ill and died within four months of each other. Together in life, they were not prepared to be parted by death. Both Jema and Donal missed them greatly. It was their first experience of death, and having to attend the two funerals of their grandparents in such a short space of time was hard for them. Donal wanted to know about heaven and if Sheila and Mossie now lived there together. I think he imagined a warm, cosy farmhouse somewhere beyond the clouds. It was a comforting vision and, even at an early age, Donal had a strong belief in an afterlife. He visited their grave with Elma and later, when he was fighting his own battle, he wrote letters to his grandparents, asking for their help and guidance. Those letters were left on their grave and he drew comfort from the belief that they were watching over him.

The Sunday afternoon drive in the summer had always included their grandparents and Elma was keen to continue the tradition of these outings, even if Sheila and Mossie were no longer with us. Usually, she took the kids to Fenit, the popular seaside village to the north of Tralee Bay, and one of Donal's favourite places. Not being content to swim from the beach, he enjoyed diving from Fenit pier into the deeper waters. Once down in the cold sea, he would try and entice Jema to join him. Not a hope!

In the swimming pool in the Tralee Leisure Centre, however, Jema was faster than her competitive brother, a situation he never managed to reverse, despite his best efforts. But he was quicker when it came to dodging the household chores which she, somehow, ended up doing while he headed off on his bike to a friend's house. When her friends called, he'd go into her bedroom without a thought and hang out with the girls. But woe betide Jema if she popped her head around his bedroom door when the boys were there! *Girls Out* was clearly the rule in force on these occasions! Like all siblings, they had their disagreements, their ups and downs, their rivalries, and yet the bond between them was forged from unconditional love.

Donal approached us one day when he was eleven and informed us that he'd decided to take up the drums. He shook his head when we – fearing the wrath of our neighbours – suggested he try the guitar or violin. No way, he said – it was the drums or nothing. It's true that it would have been difficult to imagine him sitting for hours, strumming a guitar or mastering the techniques of a violin bow. A set of drums was perfectly in character for our son, and we were not surprised by his choice.

So we bought him his first set of drums and he started drumming lessons. We also gave him the use of a small shed in the back garden, where he practised to his heart's content. Far from civilisation, we thought. But when Donal played the drums, they could be heard on the summit of Slieve Mish. Perhaps that's a slight exaggeration. Let's just say his formidable energy now had another outlet. He practised regularly and soon became quite a good drummer. He was growing fast, heading towards his teenage years and I figured it was just a matter of time before he formed his own teen band.

There are periods in life that one longs to freeze and keep that way forever – and for us, these years are one of those. As with all good times, we took them for granted and only really treasured them in retrospect. By 2008, Jema was attending secondary school and Donal was preparing to move from primary school into CBS The Green, the boys' secondary school in Tralee. So, there we were, a normal Irish family living our ordinary, contented lives. Until, overnight, our lives changed in a way we could never possibly have imagined, even in our most terrifying dreams.

Chapter Three

It began with a pain in Donal's knee. He was helping Elma clear out a shed in the back garden on the Saturday of the August weekend in 2008 when he first mentioned it. Later that evening he was playing a football match with the 'Naries' and despite the fact that the pain was still there, he headed off with Elma and Jema to take his place on the team.

The weather was balmy that evening. Enough rain had fallen throughout the summer to make a perfect backdrop for *Angela's Ashes*, but there were no clouds to worry us as Donal took up his usual position on the pitch. The game began. Donal was not the most versatile member of the team but he was taller than many of the lads, and this gave him an advantage when catching the ball. He usually played in a forward position and, although he was fiercely competitive, he was a team player and would seldom do a solo run unless he was positive he'd score. Quite often he would pass the ball to a teammate who was in a better position to take a shot at goal. But if he was in the right area of the field, he was always good for a few points or a goal or two.

He fell during the game but picked himself up and continued playing. However, some time into the second half, the pain in his knee forced him to come off the pitch. He had a strong tolerance for pain and Elma knew he was in genuine distress. He took his football seriously and he was upset as he stood on the sidelines watching the game continue. The 'Naries' won, much to his delight. Although he was usually stoic in defeat, he disliked losing and would be angry initially, especially if his team lost the game through mistakes that could have been avoided. He loved to analyse the way the game had been played: the tactics that had been employed, the build-up to a goal and so on. On this occasion his usual excitement on the way home was muted. The pain in his knee showed no sign of easing. He described it as sharp, intense and persistent.

I was managing a hotel in Dingle at the time and was on duty over the holiday weekend. Elma rang me later that night and told me about the pain Donal had been experiencing that day. She was worried. I could tell by her tone. He would never abandon a match unless he was in considerable discomfort. He'd had his share of knocks on the pitch, but he carried them lightly and looked upon them as part of the game. A few years previously he'd complained of soreness in his knee but that turned out to be a hip problem and was rectified after a short course of traction. We wondered if that problem had flared up again or if he'd taken a fall during a training session. Perhaps he had a pulled ligament, a hairline fracture or growing pains – the latter being a vague, catch-all explanation that seemed to cover a multitude of childhood aches that came and went again just as quickly … or so we believed. Our son was five feet eight inches tall, a twelve-year-old boy, growing fast. Knowing his reluctance to stay still for long periods of time, we dreaded the thought of him being confined to the sidelines until his injury healed.

That summer's holiday season was at its peak and I was busy at work. I was convinced Donal's injury would soon be sorted out. When he was a baby, he'd fallen from a changing unit. He was too small to tell us what was wrong but Elma suspected he'd hurt his arm. She took him to the doctor to see if it was fractured and, at the doctor's suggestion, Donal ate an ice cream and brought his hand to his mouth without any difficulty. He could not possibly be suffering from a fracture, the doctor decided, but the following morning, after Donal spent a fretful night crying, Elma took him to the local hospital for a check-up. An X-ray revealed a hairline fracture, and his arm was strapped up for a few weeks afterwards. Yes, I knew all about Donal's resilience to pain and I convinced myself he would be back with the 'Naries' the following weekend, playing his heart out as always.

But that was not to be the case. The following day, when the pain was still acute, Elma decided to take him to the after-hours family doctor service. An initial examination showed a build-up of fluid in his knee and some swelling. A sports-related injury was looking ever more likely. He left the clinic with a prescription for a week's supply of painkillers and anti-inflammatory tablets. But these made no difference. If anything, his knee was becoming even more painful. When I returned home a few days later, I was alarmed to notice that he was beginning to limp.

At the end of the week's treatment, Elma made an

appointment to see our regular doctor, who believed Donal could have torn tissue in his knee that had become infected and said that it could take time to heal. Donal was growing most anxious about losing his place on the team, but there was nothing he could do except wait this out. Antibiotics and more painkillers were prescribed and we strapped up his knee with a support. He was really chomping at the bit by now but he followed his doctor's instructions, hoping, like us, that every day would see an improvement.

As another fortnight passed and there was no improvement, we became increasingly anxious. Our son wasn't sleeping well and his face was drawn from the strain of this constant ache. He disliked taking painkillers – and they were only giving him an hour, or less, of relief. His limp was more pronounced now and, most alarmingly, he had no interest in going out and exercising. Unable to play or even to walk without pain upset him dreadfully. His mood veered between silence and the inevitable question: 'What do you think is wrong with my knee? *When* is it going to get better?'

We hid our anxiety and reassured him that he would soon be on the mend. We were now into the last week of August. A new school year was beginning, and Donal was starting First Year in CBS The Green. This was a new challenge – a rite of passage – and he'd been looking forward to secondary school for ages. Something urgent needed to be done. Three weeks after Donal first complained about his knee, we contacted Fionán, a family friend, who has since retired but was at the time an orthopaedic surgeon in Kerry General Hospital. Fionán sensed our panic and arranged to have the necessary X-rays done the following day. We allowed ourselves to relax a little. An X-ray would provide us with an answer and Donal's recovery process could begin.

The famous Rose of Tralee contest was being held that same week in August and, as always, the town was bustling with visitors and locals. It's always a colourful occasion, with pubs and restaurants filled to overflowing. Traffic was heavy and an air of festivity was everywhere – except, to our relief, in the A & E ward of Kerry General, where we were seen almost immediately. The X-rays were taken and examined by Fionán. We had a consultation in his office, where he informed us that there was something wrong with Donal's knee or lower thigh area. He needed an MRI scan to be done before any prognosis could be made.

An MRI sounded ominous. Fionán said he would do his utmost to get us an early appointment in a hospital in Cork, but that the public waiting list was long and we might have to wait for about two months before the scan could be done. Two months for an answer to this problem seemed a long way off. This was clearly not going to be fixed as easily as we'd originally hoped. I looked across at Elma and saw my own anxiety reflected back at me. We resigned ourselves to the fact that Donal would need intensive physiotherapy, probably traction or even an operation.

At the beginning of September, Donal dressed in his new school uniform and posed self-consciously for the obligatory first-day-at-a-new-school photograph. Then off he went to begin the second stage of his education. But after only three days' attendance at the new school, we received an unexpected phone call from our friend, Fionán. Something had been bothering him about Donal's knee and he felt it would be better to get some answers sooner rather than later. He was due to take a short break from work soon, and so he had decided to hurry the process along by organising scans the following day in the Bon Secours Private Hospital in Tralee.

This was much better. The Bon Secours is just a five-minute drive from our home and was much more convenient than the long journey to Cork. Elma arranged to be at the hospital with Donal at the agreed time the following day.

I had that afternoon off work and stayed at home to collect Jema from school. I expected Donal and Elma to be home around 4.30 p.m., with what I hoped would be a conclusive result. But instead of the car appearing in the driveway, I received a phone call from Elma. As soon as I heard her voice, I knew something was wrong. She explained that, Donal's MRI completed, they had been about to leave the Bons when she took a call on her mobile from Fionán. He had got word from the Bon Secours, and he asked her to go immediately with Donal to Kerry General Hospital for a consultation with him. More tests were needed before a definitive diagnosis could be made. I had to meet them at the Kerry General and bring a case for Donal, who would be spending the night in the children's ward. Fionán was about to leave his own home and intended stopping off at the Bons to pick up Donal's scans. He needed to speak to both of us together. I heard the urgency in Elma's voice but I still had no idea what to expect, as I began to pack my son's pyjamas and toothbrush.

I tried not to think beyond this simple chore. This was a fixable problem. It had to be fixed. Anything else was unthinkable and nothing would be served by giving way to panic. Those were my thoughts when I left the house and drove the short distance to Kerry General. Jema remained at home. She would do her homework, chat with friends on the phone, perhaps watch some television, unaware, like her parents, that we could never take anything for granted again.

Elma and Donal had arrived before me. We sat in the corridor outside the Accident and Emergency ward and waited for Fionán. We were familiar with this place. We joked with Donal, as we recalled the various emergencies that had brought us there: the time Jema drank paint thinner from a 7-Up bottle, Donal's fall from the changing unit, and other sundry accidents that had all been sorted out. This would be the same. We hid our anxiety for Donal's sake, but it was an effort to keep talking and we were relieved when we saw Fionán coming towards us along the corridor. Was he walking too fast? Was his expression concerned or relieved? Was his greeting too hearty, hiding bad news – or bringing good news? I couldn't tell. Everything was moving too quickly and we were trapped in this headlong rush. We moved into Fionán's office and waited anxiously to hear our son's prognosis.

Chapter Four

Fionán delivered the news calmly. I can only imagine the dread with which he told us that Donal's injury could be a growth, a cyst or a tumour. Was there a difference? Each word sounded equally terrifying. This was supposed to be a sports injury; growing pains; inflamed tissue. How had we suddenly moved into such dangerous territory? If I could have blocked my ears and run with my son from Fionán's office, I would have been on my feet immediately. But I needed to listen to him, to try to understand the significance of what he was telling us. Elma was rigid with shock, and Donal just looked confused, as he tried to follow Fionán's explanation.

Fionán reassured us that everything would be done as quickly as possible in order to make a definite diagnosis. His matter-of-fact approach, friendly yet professional, held us together as we absorbed each piece of new information. We had to bring Donal to Dublin, where a biopsy would be performed within the following week in Cappagh Hospital. In the meantime, Donal had to stay overnight in Kerry General so that more X-rays and tests could be done. I could see by the set of Donal's mouth that he was not enamoured of that idea. In the space of a few hours, he'd gone from what he'd believed to be a routine scan to an overnight stay in hospital. And now he was facing the prospect of an even longer stay in a strange hospital at the other side of the country. Fionán comforted him and promised to treat him like his own son but, like us, Donal must have felt as if he was on a conveyer belt that showed no sign of stopping. How had things slipped so quickly from our control?

Fionán made a point of saying that he wanted a specific chest X-ray taken. We'd no idea why, but were too stunned to ask any further questions. We had forms to fill out, arrangements with Cappagh Hospital to be made and a young, frightened boy to console. He was our main concern, and we pushed our own emotions to one side as he was checked into the Kerry General children's ward for further tests and observation. We would try to adopt Fionán's calm, matter-of-fact approach. Time enough to give way to our panic when we were alone.

I was dazed and shaken when I returned home to prepare an evening meal for Jema. I didn't want to scare her, not at this stage – or at any stage – and was non-committal when she asked why Donal was in hospital. She accepted my word, that he was undergoing some more tests on his knee and, after being reassured that he would be home the next day, she settled down to do her homework.

Elma stayed with Donal in Cashel Ward – the children's ward – until midnight and only left him when he finally fell asleep.

'What's a cyst?' he'd asked her. 'What's a biopsy?' This was a new language for him. He'd always had a close, loving relationship with his mother and Elma tried to answer him as honestly as she could. She was drained when she arrived home and could finally stop pretending that everything was going to be okay. What lay ahead for Donal, we wondered. For us as a family? To imagine our son with a cancerous growth in his knee was ludicrous. We shied away from the 'C-word', but it hung between us with all its horrifying possibilities. We could only hope and pray that the cyst was benign – but waiting for that prognosis would stretch our nerves to the limit.

Elma was back at Donal's bedside first thing the following morning, and drove him home a short while later. He was tense and worried, still asking questions, still unable to understand the enormity of what he'd been told. He wanted to return to school but the pain in his knee made that impossible.

We had tried to be as honest as possible when he asked us about the biopsy but, in reality, we had absolutely no idea what we were facing. As parents, we had age, wisdom and experience on our side. But, somehow, that was not enough. The helplessness that came from being unable to ease our son's suffering was harrowing, as we were both discovering.

On the following Thursday morning, we headed for Dublin. Cappagh Hospital is located on the outskirts of Finglas, an urban sprawl that is often in the news for all the wrong reasons. Gangland crime and drugs have taken their toll on this vibrant, hard-working community, but there was little evidence of this as we drove past the once old-fashioned village and through the vast housing estates towards the hospital's green and peaceful rural setting.

Cappagh Hospital is Ireland's highly specialised National Orthopaedic Hospital, and the friendly attitude of the staff when we arrived quickly put us at our ease. Margaret Cavanagh was the sister who would look after Donal. Fionán had praised her highly, and claimed that if there was one of her in every hospital in the country, the health service would be a whole lot more efficient – and that was some compliment, coming from him.

We were told that three doctors were waiting to examine Donal. Margaret asked Elma for the chest X-ray that Fionán had organised in Kerry General. Why Donal should need a chest X-ray had puzzled me at the time, and I now wondered why she was so anxious to see it. Elma found it in the file of scans and X-rays she'd brought with her, and handed it over. What had Donal's chest got to do with his knee? A chilling suspicion crossed my mind. What if his cancer had spread? No – I was not going there! I felt sick at the thought that this could even be considered as a possibility.

The three doctors then came to talk to Donal. Margaret told him not to hesitate if he had any questions to ask. Nothing would be kept secret from him: he would participate in all discussions and decisions about his treatment. If his medical team wished to talk to us, his parents, in private, they would ask his permission first. Our twelve-year-old son was being allowed to participate as an adult in this process. I could almost see the questions whirring around in his mind as he tried to take everything in.

Donal was shown the MRI scans of both his legs and was able

to see the comparison. His right leg showed a grey shadow of about ten centimetres in the hollow area of his knee. Grey was bad, Margaret explained as clearly and as gently as she could. But if it *was* a tumour, it would, hopefully, be benign. He listened intently as she described the difference between 'malignant' and 'benign'.

'"Benign" means that a tumour is not aggressive and doesn't spread. And then there is the other—' she paused.

'And what is the other?' he asked. 'And how will it affect me?'

She reassured him that they would only discuss that other possibility if the biopsy proved to be more serious than we all hoped. She was calm and reassuring. The fact that she was treating him as an adult and taking his questions seriously helped him to relax. She was building up a bond of trust between them, and her assurances that she would be looking after him while he was under the anaesthetic eased his fears. Margaret's manner also relieved some of our own anxieties but still, I could feel the drip, drip, drip of information taking its toll on myself and Elma. Looking back with hindsight to those early days, I can see how the process worked. We were given hope at all times, but without the possibility being completely ruled out that there could be another outcome. In a gentle, step-by-step way, we were being prepared for what could be a worst-case scenario.

The area of the bone where the cyst had developed was becoming fragile, we were told. As a precautionary measure – and to ensure he did not have more than 30 per cent of his weight on his leg in case it fractured – Donal had been given a pair of crutches soon after his arrival. He struggled to manage them as he made his way to the bathroom, and it was obvious he hated having to use them. They helped keep the pressure off his knee, but the pain persisted.

Margaret then introduced us to Mr Seán Dudeney, the surgeon who would perform the biopsy on Donal. The irony of the name was not lost on our son.

'Mr Dudeney – "do the knee", he said. In the midst of his nervousness, he was still able to laugh.

And, the consultant replied, to 'do the knee' was exactly what he intended the following morning. Had Donal any questions?

Our son nodded and the questions came tumbling out:

'How much will it hurt?'

'How big will the cut on my leg be?'

'How long will I be asleep?'

'What happens if I wake up while you're doing the biopsy?'

'What if I don't wake up afterwards?'

'How far will you drill into my thigh?'

And the question of most concern: 'How soon will I be able to eat afterwards?'

Donal was used to receiving information and absorbing it quickly. But that information usually involved him running onto a football pitch and putting what he had learned into effect there. He showed the same level of concentration as he listened to Mr Dudeney's answers. I suspected the medical personnel would soon rue the day they had allowed him such open access to information. Mr Dudeney pointed out that while he was the surgeon in charge, he only took his instructions from Margaret. She was the real boss, and Donal was to have absolute confidence in her. It was nice to see this specialist deferring authority to the person who was going to have an ongoing relationship with our son. Like everyone else who had spoken to him, Mr Dudeney was conscious of Donal's youth and the fear he was trying to hide behind all his bravado.

That evening in the ward, I soothed Donal with stories of operations I'd had when I was seven years old and, later, when I was sixteen. I'd had the same fears as he did, I told him. They were natural and understandable, but I knew, and I guess he did too, that here we were talking about something far more serious. Mr Dudeney had told us exactly how he was going to make an incision in Donal's thigh. This would be one centimetre in length, and he would then drill into the infected bone area to remove a sample for analysis. It sounded simple but of course that was no consolation to Donal, who was facing his first ever operation. He was tearful and full of fears, his misery increasing when he realised he would have to fast until after the surgery.

He kept asking about 'the Other' and Elma, like Margaret, persuaded him to stop thinking too far ahead. She would stay for the night in the hospital and I'd booked into the Skylon Hotel, which was just a short drive away. Elma finally soothed Donal to sleep while I tossed and turned and worried myself into the dawn. What if ... what if ...? It was a relief to rise early and return to the hospital to be by Donal's side as he was wheeled away.

He was, as expected, nauseous when he came round from the anaesthetic. Four hours later, he was sitting up demanding something nice to eat. Hmm, he's back, we thought, knowing from previous experiences that once his appetite returned, he was on the road to recovery. Margaret came by later and assured us they had been successful in removing a sample for analysis. There had been some difficulty, however – a vacuum in the area where there should normally be enough mass to get an easy sample. Mr Dudeney had found it slightly more difficult than expected to remove the necessary bone. This was something she had never seen before. What did that mean? Our fears reared up again. We did not want anything to be different about Donal. But Margaret seemed satisfied anyway that the sample was sufficient. We could expect results in seven to ten working days. Donal should rest for twenty-four hours and be well enough to go home with us in the morning.

The next day we returned to Blennerville to await the results. By now, our family and close friends knew we had a problem and they rallied around us, keeping us bolstered with stories of a similar nature that always ended with a successful outcome. My mother and sister, Pauline, had booked a Mediterranean cruise. We decided not to tell them how serious the situation was. They both needed a break and, we hoped, when they returned, we would have good news for them. I suggested though that when they stopped off in Rome, it would be a good idea to light a candle for Donal – and they promised to keep him in the forefront of their thoughts.

I returned to work and, over the days that followed, was only able to make it home for short periods. As the manager of a busy hotel in Dingle, I never had time to stop and think. This helped keep my fears under control during the day and it was only when I returned home that they surfaced in all their menacing power. Elma and I talked frankly about 'the Other'. It was assuming a separate identity. Something that was evil and nameless; something that breathed its unspeakable threat around us. But we were determined that none of our fears should be transferred to Donal, who had adjusted to his crutches but still hated having to use them.

'Why did this happen to me?' he kept asking. 'Why can't I be normal like my friends?'

We told him he would soon be back playing his rugby and football, back with his friends, back living the life of an active, sports-mad twelve-year-old. To imagine anything else was impossible.

I bargained with God, especially in the small hours when I was overwhelmed by dread that our son had cancer: 'Please God, if you can make sure that he's all right I will do anything – anything!' What can you promise in exchange for your child's life? I knew we could be staring into that abyss but I was not going there, not yet – not ever. And then, just as we'd psyched ourselves into the belief that all would be well, Margaret rang on 11 September 2008, with the biopsy results.

The eleventh day of September – the significance of that particular date was not lost on us, of course. Those of us who were around on that fateful day in 2001, when the Twin Towers fell to the ground, will always remember 9/11. The world was about to change. We'd no idea how this would happen or when – we just knew that change was inevitable. I was working in Dingle at the time of 9/11, and Sky News was on the television when one of the off-duty American receptionists came in to ask my permission to watch the news. She'd heard an alarming and sketchy report on the radio about a plane crashing into one of the Twin Towers. I remember looking at the pictures of the first tower, not understanding the significance of what I was seeing. Like most people, I assumed it was a tragic accident – until the second plane hit, and I realised this was something even more horrific, much more sinister. Yet it was surreal, that slow collapsing pile of bricks, glass and metal, and the silent agony of those trapped within.

Now, seven years later to the day, Elma and I were facing our own earth-shattering tragedy. A very personal tragedy of course, happening within our own family circle, but one with devastating impact and the power to utterly derail all of our lives. Elma rang me at work and broke the news. She was crying so hard, she could hardly speak. The tumour was malignant. Donal had osteosarcoma, or bone cancer as it is more commonly called. Jema was with her mother, equally distraught, as was Brian, Elma's brother. Brian was like a second father to Donal, always ready to step in as a surrogate when work took me away from home.

Once again, everything was speeding up and out of our control. Elma told me that Donal would be admitted to Our Lady's Hospital for Sick Children in Crumlin within a week. He would stay in St John's, the cancer ward, where he would begin an initial three-month programme of chemotherapy. *Chemotherapy*. I associated the term with adults – and I had seen its impact on them. Sometimes it worked and sometimes it failed. But it was always a harrowing treatment. I could not even begin to imagine how Donal was going to cope.

I left work immediately. The road from Dingle to Blennerville seemed to weave endlessly through bleak, glowering mountains, and the sea, falling below, swelled towards the shore in grey, angry waves. Everywhere I looked, I saw desolation. I knew very little about osteosarcoma, and what I did know was frightening. During my schooldays I'd been friendly with two girls who had endured amputations on their legs due to bone cancer. Both had eventually died. I hadn't thought about them in years but, now, they came vividly to mind. But that was over thirty years ago. Medicine had advanced enormously since then.

At times I had to stop the car and give way to tears. Otherwise, I would have been a danger on those twisting roads between Dingle and Blennerville. As I sat in the car at the roadside, I took phone calls from relations enquiring about the biopsy results and, somehow, I managed to speak sensibly to them. I heard that pause when I told them, the intake of breath or shocked exclamation, the sadness in their voices as they did their best to comfort me.

The white sails of the Blennerville Windmill came into view. I had to drive across the bridge to reach my home. My family were waiting on the other side. I needed to be composed when they saw me. I tried to imagine what words Elma and I would use to tell Donal our worst fears had come to pass. No such words came to mind but, somehow, we all had to find the courage to face what lay ahead.

Chapter Five
Donal's Story

The first time they told me, I was at home – I was on the phone to my friend. It was 11 September 2008. My mom came in, she didn't have to say anything, I knew straight away what had happened: the test results were bad and the tumour was malignant. I hung up the phone without saying anything and I felt like throwing it at the wall. But to be honest, I didn't know what it meant. I was twelve, and all I cared about was playing sport. I knew it was bad but I didn't understand the severity of it. I had cancer, a tumour that had grown on my right femur just above my knee, and little did I know it would destroy parts of my life that I had never planned on letting go of.

Chapter Six

'The Other' had ceased to be a shadow and was now our reality. Initially, when cancer invades your home, you are bereft of words. Your thoughts are in turmoil. Your body wants to close down and sleep, until you can wake up and realise you were dreaming your worst nightmare. There is no way to avoid it. No fork in the road, offering you the choice of a different path to the one you are now on. But, gradually, as your mind accepts the unbelievable, you have to muster all your strength and deal with what has been placed before you.

Donal was shocked and upset – and angry too. In his writings, we see that confusion. He was too young to understand the gravity of his illness, and his main annoyance was that he would miss the early months in his new school and not be able to play football. It worried him that his friends would make new friends and forget about him. He had to hang around the house when Jema left for school, and it all seemed so unfair to our super-active twelve-year-old son. But he quickly accepted the changes that had to come. He was anxious for the treatment to start, so that he could be cured and return to his real life as soon as possible.

We too were beginning to come to grips with the news. Decisions had to be made. Elma, anticipating what lay ahead, gave up her job. Her employer was understanding and supportive. Her position would remain open until Donal was cured and she could return to the company. Jema's routine also had to be considered. She too was dealing with the shock of her brother's illness but, as with Donal, we tried to cushion her from the harsh facts. Brian, as always, stepped into the breach and agreed to move into the house to look after her while we were in Dublin. I arranged to take six weeks off work, so that I could be with Donal and Elma through the various stages of his treatment.

Elma and I had made a conscious decision to go public with the news in our immediate circles. Donal's young friends from school, and those in the rugby and football clubs, needed to be prepared. Once his chemotherapy began, his appearance would change dramatically. They needed to appreciate that, while they would see physical changes in him, he would still be the same person they had always known. Telling Mary, Donal's grandmother on my side, was going to be difficult. She adored Donal and I knew she would be devastated when she returned from her cruise. To help me break the news to her, I drew on the support of her brother – my uncle, Bill Morrison, who lives in Dublin – and my own brother Michael, who is a priest. We met her and my sister Pauline in Bewley's hotel at Dublin airport on the morning after their return. I guess they must have known as soon as they saw our faces. But my mother is a strong woman, and she did not falter as she absorbed the enormity of what I had to tell her. Support was coming in waves from family and friends. We were astonished and buoyed up by people's generosity – and the support offered to us was both moral and financial. As yet, we hadn't realised the financial implications of Donal's illness and were more concerned with making his few remaining days at home before going to Crumlin as enjoyable as possible.

I made two particular calls to rugby colleagues and told them about our situation. One of these colleagues was Martin, who had contacts with the Ronald McDonald House (RMDH), which is based in the grounds of Crumlin Hospital. It was set up to provide accommodation to those who have to travel from afar and want to stay with their sick children, who are undergoing treatment in Crumlin. As well as offering accommodation, the aim of the charity is to create a supportive, caring environment for such families. Donal would be spending three weeks of each month in Dublin. I asked Martin how we could gain access to this facility. The journey from our home in Tralee to Dublin takes about three-and-a-half hours, so a base near the hospital was clearly essential. We were promised rooms as soon as they became available and, thankfully, we did not have long to wait before we received word that we could be accommodated.

The second call I made was to Dave, the Ticket Manager at Tralee RFC, to cancel all the tickets I'd booked for the Munster matches that year. Instead, I wanted just one thing: a dream ticket for the contest of the century – Munster versus the All Blacks – which was to be held in November. No matter what the treatment, no matter what the timing – even if I had to take Donal out of hospital for the day and drive him down to Thomond Park and stand outside during the match, then return him to the hospital afterwards – he was going to be there. Thirty years earlier, on that unforgettable day when Munster won their historic victory over the All Blacks, I had not been present in Thomond to celebrate. But now, thirty years later, my son was not going to miss out on this opportunity. Dave promised to do everything he could to grant my request.

On the Friday of that week when Donal was still at home, Jay Galvin, a friend and member of Tralee RFC, phoned and asked if Donal could be at the rugby club around 7 p.m. that evening. A special 'surprise' visitor had arrived and he was anxious to meet Donal. Jay gave us no further information, but the thought of meeting this mysterious visitor was enough to lift Donal's mood. The 'why me?' questions had started in earnest since he heard the results of the biopsy. He had shed many bewildered tears over the days which followed, but I saw his eyes brighten when he heard that a 'special' visitor was very keen to meet him. We all tried to guess who it was, but were no wiser as we set off for the club. What a surprise when we arrived and discovered that Paul O'Connell, a giant on and off the rugby pitch, was waiting for us!

Paul, who was captaining Munster at the time, had come

to Tralee to give our senior players a training session. News of Donal's diagnosis had spread among the members and Paul, when he heard that he was Donal's hero, had asked to be introduced to him. I know that Paul O'Connell needs no introduction to anyone who knows anything about rugby. He's an integral member of the Ireland and Munster teams. He'd led Munster to their second Heineken Cup victory in May of that year at the Millennium Stadium in Cardiff, where they beat French team Toulouse 16–13. Donal had watched the Heineken final, cheering the triumphant team all the way, and now couldn't believe his good fortune when his hero spent time talking to him and posing for photographs. Paul chose that evening to meet him at the club in Tralee, knowing that on the following day, when he'd arranged to greet the underage teams, Donal would be swallowed up in the melee of young, excited fans. Donal's eyes were shining with pride and excitement as he stood beside Paul, unaware that this was the beginning of a friendship that would see him through every stage of his illness.

I am convinced that the human body reacts to positive experiences. I cannot emphasise this enough. Donal's meeting with Paul was the first of many positive events we and others would organise for him over the following months. Anything that would energise him or give him goals to achieve would be used as part of his treatment. We were under no illusions as to what lay ahead. His competitive nature would be called upon to fight the biggest battle of his young life and he would need to draw on all the psychological strengths he'd learned on the training ground and surround himself with positivity. Poison was about to be infused into his system to kill this disease but his soul needed therapy as well – and such incentives would be an important aspect of his recovery.

Chapter Seven

On this high note, Donal headed for Dublin and Our Lady's Hospital for Sick Children. He'd developed the MRSA bug, which he'd probably contracted during one of his hospital visits or he could just as easily have picked it up on the street. There are a lot of myths out there about MRSA but, realistically, anyone, whether in hospital or not, can be a carrier without being infected – and Donal, although not infected, was carrying the bug. Due to the vulnerability of the patients in the cancer ward, he would remain in isolation until three clear nasal swabs showed that all traces had gone from his system.

In a way, this period of isolation was a relief, as it eased us more gently into the routine of the hospital. Three busy days of tests followed, along with meetings with oncologists, social workers, treatment planners, dieticians, home treatment advisors, nurses, physiotherapists and medical trainers. A mystifying and highly complex new world was opening up before us, and we were on a sharp learning curve.

Dr Capra, the consultant oncologist who would be looking

after Donal, and his two residents – Chris from Nigeria and Owen from Ireland – introduced themselves and gave us the details of Donal's programme for the next few days: tests, scans and checks on the various functions of his body in its pre-chemotherapy state. In this way they would be able to assess him as he went through the treatment process, and see if there were any significant changes. The tests included liver, kidney and aural examinations, as well as scans to see if there was more than one point of infection – or, as they put it, 'secondary tumours'. *Secondary* tumours? This immediately brought to mind that chest X-ray and its sinister implications. The possibility that our son's cancer had spread terrified us. But we could not receive this information until all Donal's tests had been completed. The medical team meeting would be held that Thursday and so, from Monday onwards, we lived in this state of limbo, awaiting these results.

On Wednesday afternoon Donal got a respite from the tests and was allowed out of hospital for a few hours. We toured the Dundrum Shopping Centre. He'd always enjoyed shopping for clothes but on this occasion he was more interested in buying a camera.

'I want to take photographs of all that's going to happen to me from now on,' he said.

I could see subtle changes in him. His earlier shock and anger had gone and this new challenge he was facing was taking on the proportions of a match final, from which he intended to emerge victorious. No medals this time, just his old life back again. The camera he bought became one of his most important possessions over the following months, and was used to record the many experiences he had on his road to recovery. After this purchase, he was anxious to eat. He would lose his taste for food with the onset of chemotherapy and this would be his last opportunity to enjoy a wholesome meal for some time to come. Donal never adjusted to hospital food – it wasn't home cooking and, as such, was endured rather than enjoyed. After our meal, it was back to the hospital, and the spectre of our appointment with the medical team on the following day settled upon us once again.

The next morning, preparations for the chemotherapy began. This involved the installation of a Hickman line – known to the children on the ward as a 'Freddie line' – into Donal's chest. This would lead up to his neck and into his jugular vein. His medical team would be able to take continuous blood tests and to medicate him without having to stick needles into him each time. To have the Hickman line installed, Donal had to undergo minor surgery, and he was put to sleep once again.

While he was under the anaesthetic Elma and I attended a meeting with Dr Capra and Fiona, the liaison nurse. It began in the calm, professional way that was by now becoming familiar to us. We were given details of the treatment they would use and its effects on Donal. We were then presented with the options that could follow Donal's first three months of chemotherapy. The chemotherapy would shrink the tumour and, when this was achieved, one of these three courses of action would be decided upon. Each one sounded grim and unbelievably difficult.

The first option: a section of Donal's thigh would be removed and rebuilt. This procedure could take a number of years to complete, and could only be done in the first place if the tumour had shrunk sufficiently.

The second option: if the growth of the tumour had reached the area of his knee that was still growing, this would necessitate a larger section of Donal's lower thigh being removed and replaced with a prosthetic.

The third – and worst – option: the removal of the lower limb from above the tumour. In other words, full amputation.

As yet, we had no idea which option would be chosen. I broke down in tears and wept uncontrollably. Our son, the rugby player, the footballer, the athlete – would he be able to walk properly again? And even if he could, would he ever be able to run?

It seemed, in those early weeks, as if Elma and I were being hit by a train, not just once but continuously, each blow harder than the last. We were utterly devastated and could only imagine the terror Donal would experience when this momentous decision would eventually be made. Dr Capra allowed me to weep my fill, then reminded me that my tears were no use to Donal. They would deplete his energy and determination as he underwent his battle. We had to be as positive and as courageous as he was. As his parents, that was our responsibility.

We were still waiting to hear about test results that would confirm whether or not Donal had a secondary tumour. Finally, towards the end of the meeting, Elma found the courage to ask the dreaded question. Only then were we told that the cancer was confined to Donal's lower thigh area. How can I describe the pent-up tension we'd struggled to contain while waiting for such news? The relief was so physical, I didn't know whether to throw up or offer up a prayer of thanksgiving. That we should feel such relief because our son did not have secondary tumours was a frightening indication of how far our mindset had shifted since we heard that first terrifying prognosis.

And so we began our journey into Donal's hell.

Chapter Eight
Donal's Story

The first chemotherapy started on 18 September 2008. Before that, I was in so much pain, I had gone weeks with only hours of sleep and countless different medications. But nothing would stop it. In a way, I'm glad the painkillers didn't work. If they had, I wouldn't have said anything, the pain would have disappeared and the cancer spread, and I might not have had the same outcome that I was given. Even to this day, I refuse painkillers, not because I'm stupid but because I'm afraid. I'm afraid if I cover it up that it could be serious and by the time I realise it, it might be too late.

Amazingly, when they started chemo, the pain stopped. A good sign: it was working. Doxorubicin, cisplatin and methotrexate were my chemotherapies. They were my best friends and my worst enemies. They would save my life and nearly kill me. But I was doing it. I wanted to live, to play for Munster, to travel the world, to raise children and die when I'm a hundred, not twelve.

I had a lot of bad days over the next few weeks. I was going downhill fast and everyone knew it. Everyone except me. I couldn't see what was happening to me, I would walk into the hospital for my chemo, take my bed next to a baby – I'd see two adults asleep on the floor. I'd take my vomiting bowl and pee jar for the week. Then I'd sleep. I shut it out. I didn't want to be like the three-year-olds who would walk around with smiles and buckets of toys. I wanted to be Donal. But when you walk in there, you lose everything – your pride, your dignity and, once they start the chemo, you lose your body. In a way, the smaller children have an easier path. They won't remember this. But it's harder for their parents because they have to watch this happen to their children.

Normality changes too. I had trouble struggling to figure out what it was for me. I'd wake up and get my injection, I'd get sick a couple of times a day, I'd wander around the house, waiting for school to finish and maybe a few friends would come over. They didn't treat me the same. I was different: I was that person you stop your kids from staring at. I was sick.

Chapter Nine

Everyone we knew was anxious to do something to make Donal's time in St John's Ward a little easier. Despite the effects of the chemo on his system, he was determined to enjoy the build-up to the All-Ireland Football Final towards the end of September, when Kerry would play Tyrone. Eileen and Tom, close friends of our family, organised a Get Well Soon card to be signed for Donal by the players on the Kerry team. Donal knew them all by reputation, and reading a card with their names on it cheered him up no end. An added bonus was the parcel that came with it. When he opened it, he found a jersey from Tommy Walsh – the one Tommy wore in the semi-final when he scored his first senior goal in Croke Park. Donal was thrilled to receive this and wore it during the All Ireland Final.

Sadly, it was not Kerry's day. They were defeated by Tyrone and the following day – when the victorious Tyrone team followed the usual tradition and visited the children in Crumlin Hospital to show off the famous Sam Maguire cup – Donal, wearing his Tommy Walsh jersey, welcomed them into his room, which was bedecked in the gold and green colours of the Kerry team. There was much good-natured slagging between him and the team about the match. Regretfully, he waved goodbye to the Sam Maguire as it was carried in triumph over the border to Northern Ireland. But he was convinced it would be back in 'the Kingdom' the following year.

This was one of the good days in the midst of what, to Donal, must have seemed like a waking nightmare. I remained in Dublin for those first six weeks of his treatment and Elma became his chief carer. She learned quickly and soon became familiar with the different cancer terms. She understood what each treatment did and how it would affect Donal. He questioned everything, as we had told him to do, and Elma was able to impart all the relevant information to him. She was shown how to do dressings and injections, how to clean the tubes that infused the chemo into his system. His hospital ward became a cocoon, the world outside a distant place with unrelated cares. Sometimes, emerging from the hospital environs, Elma and I would blink at the noise of traffic and the rush of fresh air on our faces. We'd look at the pedestrians hurrying by, blissfully unaware of that other world behind those walls, where life and death rubbed shoulder to shoulder, and patients, family and staff formed a close-knit community. Neither the patients nor their families had ever planned on joining this community but, now that we had, we were immediately absorbed into the bustling tempo of the hospital.

We could not afford to stay in hotels or rent accommodation for a long period of time. Our relations in Dublin were more than generous when it came to providing accommodation, but we needed to be as close to Donal as possible. As soon as a room became available, the Ronald McDonald House became our home from home. On our arrival, we were greeted by Mairéad, the house manager, her staff and the volunteers, and were allocated one of the sixteen rooms with private bathroom facilities. In the public areas we had access to a play room and library, a small garden, a TV room and a laundry. Three kitchens led into the communal dining facility. We were allocated a separate fridge, freezer and dry goods storage area so that our food was secure and separated from other residents. It was a tremendous relief to be able to rely on this marvellous facility and it was here, in the RMDH, that we came to appreciate that Crumlin was a children's hospital and not just a cancer unit. We met parents of children of all ages, from newborn infants to teenagers, who had many different ailments.

As we listened to other people's stories, we came to realise, in relative terms, that Donal was fortunate, in that he had only one tumour and a strong chance of a full recovery at the end of his torturous journey. Other families were living on the flimsiest thread of hope that their child would survive the following twenty-four hours.

At the other end of the scale, I met a mother whose child had severe tonsillitis. This was when Donal was in the throes of chemotherapy. As far as this mother was concerned, her child's situation was traumatic and extreme, and she was highly stressed over it. I've no doubt however that if she was faced with a greater trauma, her shoulders would broaden and she would find the backbone she needed. We do not know our coping abilities until we are challenged and discover an inner strength we never knew existed.

Occasionally celebrity chefs or the chefs from local restaurants came and cooked a meal for the residents of the house. Sometimes, they were just volunteers with no prior catering experience who provided wholesome, delicious food for up to sixty people. Being in the hotel industry, I'd a keen awareness of the organisation and preparation this entailed. But, most importantly, these communal meals created the opportunity for a social gathering for the parents and guardians who barely had time to talk to each other as their duty-shifts changed. We were like ships passing in the night. All of us hoping that a safe harbour lay ahead.

Chapter Ten

By the beginning of October Donal had completed his first three weeks of chemo and was beginning to lose his hair. He would have expected to worry about the occasional pimple or greasy skin as he entered puberty – not the loss of his hair. The prospect horrified him, especially as he would also lose his eyebrows and the hair that had started to grow in his pubic region. He was at home on his week off when Elma noticed the first signs. She would casually brush the hairs from his shoulders or hoover them from the floor. He had a thick head of dark hair and, at first, he was unaware it had started to happen. But it was only a matter of time before it became noticeable.

Jon Kenny, a friend who had survived cancer twice, agreed to meet Donal for a man-to-man talk about some of the effects he would be likely to experience from the chemotherapy.

He cheerfully reassured Donal that all his hair would grow back within six weeks of ending his treatment. This appeased Donal – but only slightly. Jon then said that the most important thing he could get was a pair of long johns, as the loss of hair on his legs would mean that he'd feel the cold there more than usual. Practical advice delivered with humour: this was exactly what Donal needed. Before they parted, they exchanged phone numbers and Jon gave him a picture of the Irish rugby team playing against their fiercest rivals, England, in that historic match at Croke Park on 24 February 2007. Ireland had won that day and Donal would win his battle with cancer, said Jon. He also invited us to join him at the Munster v Glasgow Warriors match in the new Thomond Park on the following Saturday. I believed at the time that we would be unable to go, as Donal might be too weak from his treatment. But I changed my mind when things took a dramatic turn for the worse.

It was indeed a very dark day for our family when I received a call from Margaret in Cappagh Hospital, who told me that a decision had been made on one of the three options open to Donal when he finished his chemotherapy. He was to have part of his knee and thigh removed and a prosthesis inserted. This operation would be carried out in the New Year in Cappagh Hospital and performed by Mr Dudeney. *Do the knee ... Do the knee ...* This manic thought ran through my mind as I remembered Donal joking about it before the biopsy, when we still had hope.

Margaret asked if Donal could come to Dublin a day earlier than his next planned visit to Crumlin, and stay overnight in Cappagh Hospital, so that scans could be done for this prosthesis. *Whoa there, Margaret,* I thought. *Hold back a little and give me time to breathe.* We were supposed to have had three options under consideration. Why had the second option been chosen so quickly? Margaret's response was sympathetic but practical. Scans had revealed that the tumour had reached a crucial area of Donal's knee and this therefore necessitated the removal of a section of his lower thigh.

Osteosarcoma is the most common form of bone cancer and can occur early in the teen years, when children are experiencing a growth spurt. Boys are more likely to develop osteosarcoma than girls, and one of the symptoms is swelling of the knee. Our twelve-year-old son, tall for his age and long-boned, was a classic example. His knee had swollen, pained him at night and caused him to limp. Now, the cancerous area would be removed and Donal would have to learn to walk again. I felt weak as I listened to this bleak prognosis.

January was still over three months away. Why the rush with the scans? Margaret informed me that it would take time for the prosthesis to be made in Stanmore in London, where they are produced. Each prosthesis is made to very specific and individual measurements. Donal was a growing boy, and the prosthesis would be designed to accommodate his growth. Work had to begin immediately to ensure it was a perfect fit and capable of being adjusted when necessary. I ended the call, wondering how on earth I was going to break the news to Elma and Donal. He had been aware of these options but I don't believe he fully understood the significance of what lay ahead, no matter which one was chosen. I called Elma's brother Brian and filled him in on what was happening. He agreed to take Donal out for a drive, while I sat down with Elma to discuss this catastrophic turn of events. Donal was to have major surgery in January – surgery that would alter his life forever.

Elma's shock mirrored my own. There were tears, of course, many of them. But with our tears came resignation. It was not the worst of the three options, and we were learning to be thankful for small mercies. By the time Donal and Brian arrived back, we had composed ourselves but, inwardly, we were still sobbing as we prepared to break the news to our son. Normally, when our children were sick in bed, we could hold them and comfort them through their pain. We could lower their temperatures, soothe their headaches, be there when they called us. But this was different. Donal was in the hands of strangers – compassionate and caring strangers, admittedly – and now they were the ones in control.

Chapter Eleven
Donal's Story

I had one of the worst days of my life. My uncle took me out for a drive. I wasn't eating again. I didn't eat after chemo. I couldn't, I didn't have an appetite at all and anything I did eat wouldn't be long in my stomach before it was in the vomiting bowl.

When we came home, I was told to sit down. They told me that I would need surgery and it was more complicated than they thought. It was too close to my knee for bone salvage surgery, so they would need to remove half my femur, all my knee and a small part of my tibia and replace it with prosthetics. I knew what this meant: sport was gone. My dream, the only thing I wanted, was gone. I was devastated. I couldn't talk to anyone for days.

Chapter Twelve

When Donal heard the news, he was as devastated as we had anticipated. We remembered the advice we'd received from Dr Capra and did our utmost to be strong and hide our fears from him. A positive approach was the only way forward. And so we focused on looking at the advantages of this operation. It was not as drastic as an amputation and his recovery would be faster than with the first option, which could have taken a number of years to complete. Donal remained silent and withdrawn for a few days, but I could see him slowly pulling himself together. I contacted Jon Kenny to see if the tickets for the Munster v Glasgow Warriors game were still available. They were, and Jon was delighted that we could join him. We would have access to the supporters' lounge and Donal would have a chance to see his hero Paul O'Connell again.

On the morning of the match, he woke and found the first really large clump of hair on his pillow. He struggled not to cry but the sight was too much for him. He was still only a twelve-year-old boy and, in a week of bad news, this was the final straw. The hair loss wasn't really noticeable to anyone but himself, yet nothing would convince him otherwise. He shed anguished tears and declared that he would not go to Thomond Park where, he was convinced, everyone would stare at him. He only calmed down when I brought him to the bathroom mirror and showed him that the loss wasn't as obvious as he believed. In the end he put his worries to one side and by the time we reached Thomond Park, the excitement of the occasion took over.

Jon had invited us to dine at his table before the match. We were accompanied by Michael, my brother, and Bill, my uncle. Thomond Park had undergone a huge renovation. This was the first official game in the new stadium and the unofficial opening of the venue to a capacity crowd. We enjoyed our food before the match, received a briefing from the Munster coaches, some light entertainment and then the game itself. Out came Donal's camera, along with his smile. He took some amazing photographs, in particular one of Ronan O'Gara kicking off the first ball of the match.

Throughout the match I kept thinking of all the rugby matches my son had played and the matches he would never get to play in the future. All contact sports would have to be avoided once his prosthesis was in place. I thought of how, hail, rain or snow, Donal had always practised his drop-kicking for an hour each day. A second-row forward doesn't need to practise place or drop-kicking, but Donal did. He'd always wanted to play the number 10 out-half position and had, on one occasion, drop-kicked a goal to win the game. His coach told him in no uncertain terms that second-row forwards were not supposed to do that, but two weeks later, to Donal's delight, a Glaswegian prop forward did exactly the same in the Magners League, a feat which also won the match. And so Donal had continued to practise his drop-kicking, curving the ball around the house so that it didn't go into our neighbour's garden *all* the time. Little did I realise, as I watched him practise, how his determination and discipline would have such a profound influence on him when illness struck and it seemed as if an entire opposing team was intent on taking him down.

As the match progressed, Donal started to tug at his hair. It came out in small clumps, not really noticeable until he showed me what he was doing. I was afraid he was going to break down and cry again but, instead, he dropped the clumps of hair to the ground.

'Well, Dad, now there's a little bit of me in Thomond Park,' he said, and then I was the one who felt like howling.

Munster were victorious and the excitement continued when the match was over. In the supporters' lounge we enjoyed the triumphant atmosphere. The anticipation mounted when the team arrived. When Paul O'Connell saw Donal, he invited him to join the team at their table for the post-match meal. I was put on camera duty to take as many pictures as I could of Donal with the Munster legends. He was sitting between Anthony ('Axel') Foley and Paul O'Connell, when the latter called Ronan O'Gara over to join them. Ronan sat beside Donal and asked what was wrong with his leg. He was genuinely interested in hearing about Donal's cancer. I was amazed to hear Donal relate the complex details of his tumour and his treatment – and Ronan was equally practical with his questions and comments.

Donal was flushed with excitement, thrilled to be in the presence of his heroes. By being able to discuss his condition with those he admired, everything that awaited him back at the hospital seemed more manageable, and would, somehow, be endured.

We headed straight back to Tralee, exhausted but elated. We promised to return to this field of dreams as soon, and as often, as possible over the coming year. After the excitement of the day, Donal slept for most of the journey home. He then recounted the details to Elma and Jema, with a veritable scrapbook of photos to show them.

A clump of his hair remained on the terraces when we left that evening and, even if the wind blew it away, I knew that Donal carried with him the fighting spirit of Thomond Park.

But his hair loss was tough on him, and the bravery he had shown in Thomond Park was difficult to maintain. He was angry and distraught every time he examined himself in the mirror or saw fresh clumps on his pillow. But there was nothing he could do about it and, once the shock receded, he started dealing with it in his usual resolute manner. When, after another bout of chemo, it began to fall out in earnest, he shaved it off and started wearing a beanie hat.

The hat made its first public appearance when he attended his under-12 football team's county semi-final. At first he'd been reluctant to go, convinced his friends would be put off by the changes in him. But eventually we persuaded him to come with us, plus his camera. Once he arrived at the pitch, he became energised. He had to cope with the fact that he was now standing on the sidelines, knowing that he would never again take to the field with his teammates. But he took his photographs and was able to record the victory of the 'Naries' against Mitchells.

Donal might have been able to hide his hair loss but he was becoming progressively dependent on the crutches. The expressions of sympathy and concern from all his friends, and their parents, were overwhelming. But I was keenly aware too that the parents were now looking at the injuries and growing pains of their own children in a different light. Our only relief was that the cancer had not spread or 'metastasised' – another new word that was becoming familiar – to his lungs or other bones. A neighbour of ours told me later that she had been amazed by my composure when I told her that Donal had cancer in *only* one area. After I'd explained the danger of his cancer spreading, she was able to appreciate the mental journey Elma and I had taken to reach that awareness and manage to be grateful for it.

With each visit home from the hospital, Donal tried to attend any training session or game in both rugby and football. But these trips were becoming less frequent as his condition deteriorated.

By now, the beanie hat was achieving the status of a fashion item. Once he knew a friend was calling on his or her first visit since he had begun losing his hair, he would wear the hat for half an hour after his or her arrival. 'I don't want to scare them off with the baldness,' he said. 'When they get used to seeing that I'm still me, the Donal they know, then I'll take it off.'

I was impressed by his desire not to cause discomfort to these young people. They had no idea of what Donal was going through for three weeks out of every month, and Donal wanted to keep it that way. He now had two lives. In hospital, he was a patient. At home, he was Donal and had no wish to discuss his illness with us, Jema or any of his friends.

As October drew to a close, his treatment was becoming more aggressive. He hated the train trip to Dublin to begin a fresh round of chemo. On one occasion he stood on the platform in Tralee station and refused to board the train. He'd had enough, he told Elma. But he gave in, just as the train was about to leave, and another session began.

Apart from his hair, his weight loss was showing, and the nausea and vomiting were more frequent as he grew weaker after each chemotherapy session. The medical team were worried about his weight loss and discussed the possibility of introducing a nasal tube. Donal flatly refused to consider this option. He was cooperating fully with everything he was being asked to do, but he balked at this. Somehow, to him, it would emphasise his helplessness in his fight against his cancer. For all of us, the cancer had assumed a separate identity. It had become an alien force that had invaded his system and our lives. When we vented our anger, it was directed solely at this voracious disease. We supported Donal in his refusal to have a nasal tube inserted. As long as he was eating well in between treatments, we were getting some stability on his weight. A decision was made to put him on a food supplement. He hated it. We tried to disguise it in his food but he had the instincts of a bloodhound and would instantly know we'd tampered with what he was eating. We were more successful with pancakes, which he'd always liked, and when he was home, his breakfast consisted of a plate of pancakes, laced with supplements, but carefully disguised with lemon juice and other tasty accompaniments.

We were proud of how he was handling each setback that came his way, but how we wished our pride was based on something else – anything other than the maturity he was gaining through his suffering. He was becoming too wise for his tender years, and our hearts were breaking for him.

Chapter Thirteen

But what of Jema during this tumultuous time? She had been keeping a brave face on things and we assumed she was coping with the long periods of time Elma and I were spending in Dublin. Brian continued to act in loco parentis during those times but, even when we were at home for a week at the end of each three-week chemo session, our focus was on Donal.

The first realisation that Jema might not be coping as well as we thought came when we saw how her subject grades had dropped during her mid-term examinations. We should not have been surprised. The family routine she had always taken for granted must have looked like it was falling apart. We'd tried to protect her from the reality of Donal's illness but in protecting her, we'd only added to her bewilderment. We were in the midst of a storm and it was difficult to hold on to each other when the winds were blowing us this way and that. We needed to talk to Jema about her grades and try to get her back on track.

Her reaction, when we finally had this discussion, left us in no doubt about how she felt. She was frantic with worry over Donal, she said, yet we expected her to cope on her own and carry on as if everything was normal. It wasn't – and all we wanted her to do was achieve good grades! Her outburst pulled us up short and made us realise how affected she was by our deep-rooted, unspoken fears, and the tense atmosphere these created.

Fortunately, around this time, Catriona Goggin, the social work team leader for paediatrics in Kerry General Hospital, came into our lives and helped us concentrate on the issues facing us – and to understand the loneliness of the 'Other Child or Children,' who can so easily be left out of the loop. Donal was at the centre of our conversations and our prayers, and constantly on our minds. We could not control his pain, but we could make his days as enjoyable as possible under these grim circumstances. So he had his treats and outings – and our entire attention also. Donal's illness had consumed us all and Jema was forced to look on from the sidelines, with no idea what was going on when we were in hospital with him.

Catriona was able to give us some sound advice about how to deal with an issue we'd been aware of but had been too preoccupied to address. Everyone in our family was affected by Donal's cancer and this included Jema, who should always be included in family discussions. She needed to know we loved her as much as we always had, and that her concerns – however minor they might seem compared to what Donal was enduring – were important to us. Put quite simply, she needed us to slow down and put our arms around her.

We worked out a new regime. I went to Dublin with Donal for the first few days of each treatment, then swapped duties with Elma midweek. Donal could then finish his treatment and go to the Ronald McDonald House with his mother for his few free days before he had to return for his next bout of chemotherapy. This way, at least one parent would be at home while the other did bedside duty with Donal.

The hotel where I worked was now closed for the winter season. On those days when I was at home, I'd drop Jema to school, go directly to the hotel, update all the computers, input any information required and be home in time to collect her, cook her dinner and help with her studies. We were very fortunate to have the support of Erica Healy, a family friend who helped Jema with grinds and became her confidante throughout Donal's illness. Erica understood how tough things were for Jema and would organise visits to the cinema and other outings to keep her spirits up. We were all feeling our way through this tumultuous time and if Jema had questions she was afraid to ask us for fear of adding to our stress, we could now hear about them through another source.

By November 2008, after two months of chemotherapy, the effects on Donal were obvious. His weight loss was more evident, the nausea and vomiting more frequent. He'd lost his hair and the beanie cap was worn most of the time now. When he came home during his week off from chemotherapy, I learned to administer his daily injection. I found this increasingly difficult to do. There was so little fatty tissue on his body and he'd have severe bruising after each shot. I had to learn to inject with only the minimum needle pressure, so that I didn't hit a vein.

He developed a cough and the strain of constantly coughing caused him to vomit. We tried to organise a medicine that would give him some relief, but his treatment was so finely balanced that anything extra would destabilise his blood levels. In the end he was only allowed to use Ventolin. This eased the effects but did not get rid of his cough. He so badly needed another bright spot on his horizon. Once again, rugby would provide the answer.

We'd received confirmation that the tickets were in the bag for the upcoming match between Munster and the All Blacks that November. And Donal's excitement was high as the date of the match drew nearer.

Chapter Fourteen

On the Sunday before the match, some of the All Blacks team had officially opened the Munster Museum in Thomond Park. Supporters were welcome so, needless to say, we made the pilgrimage. Tom, Donal's uncle, was in charge of the sound equipment and we were able to stand inside the restriction barriers. I also made sure to find out where I could park my car the following Tuesday night when the match would take place. Donal's leg would not permit long walks or queuing. I'd sought out the head of security, who gave me his card and offered us easy access to the stadium. Again, strangers came to our rescue and became friends.

Finally, on the big day – 18 November 2008 – we arrived in Thomond Park about two hours prior to the game. Donal wolfed down his hot dog and chips. What a relief to get away for once from food supplements and the strict hospital diet! We attended the match with Brian and my uncle, Bill. Their kindness at this difficult time will never be forgotten and they made a terrific fuss of Donal, who was wearing his beanie hat and had his camera at the ready.

Munster were prepared for this challenge against the most formidable opposition in world rugby. And they had a heavy mantle to carry, if they were to live up to the reputation of their predecessors from thirty years earlier. We took our places in the west stand to the resounding beat of the Munster Army Drummers. The excitement continued to build as both teams went through their warm-up rituals. Afterwards, the drummers lined up at the entrance, as the then Taoiseach, Brian Cowen, formally opened the redeveloped Thomond Park. The heroes of the 1978 victory were then presented to the crowd, who applauded them rapturously. A light from the city end of the stadium appeared in the clear night sky and hovered above us. It grew bigger, wider and illuminated the pitch. Then, to the delight of the crowd, two members of the Irish Air Force abseiled down from a helicopter into the centre of the pitch, with the match ball. The tension was building rapidly and when the drummers intensified their beat, the crowd responded with a mighty roar. At last, the teams appeared, and Donal was cheering as loudly and as wildly as anyone else in the crowd.

Rumour had gone around the stadium that something special was going to happen before the game. The Munster team linked arms and lined up to accept the Haka from the All Blacks – or so we believed. Then, to the utter delight and cheers of support from the crowd, our four Munster players from the southern hemisphere – Dougie Howlett, Justin Melck, Rua Tipoki and Lifeimi Mafi – stepped forward and proceeded to do a Haka of welcome for the All Blacks. The gauntlet had been thrown down! After the cheering died away, the All

Blacks responded with their own Haka, to a respectful silence from everyone in the stadium. Anyone who knows rugby and has visited Thomond Park understands what a respectful silence means in that stadium. This silence is so complete that you will hear the bleep of a text on a mobile phone, even if you are in the opposite stand. The ending of the Haka was greeted with a lusty roar from the crowd and then the chants of, 'Munster, Munster!' These visitors were under no illusion they were visitors, and were now in the centre of the cauldron that is Thomond Park.

The Munster team were buoyed up by this support. They knew they had to play out of their skins on this night of all nights. And that was what they did. Bodies were thrown on the line to ensure that the All Blacks knew that they had come to the spiritual home of Irish rugby. I looked over at Donal several times during the game. His crutches were abandoned and he was leaping from his seat, roaring in support of his heroic Munster team or shouting against a perceived wrongdoing by the opposition. Impossible to believe he had a tumour in his leg or that he was deep in the maelstrom of chemotherapy.

All of history will debate the penalty given to the All Blacks against the Munster captain, Mick O'Driscoll – but this led to the final try by the visitors. Sadly, that won the game for them, by 18–16. No one could have expected more from this Munster team. With their battle-worn demeanour, they would not have looked out of place in a hospital emergency room. Exhaustion, cramp and aching muscles were being suffered all over the pitch, but the Munster men had fought brilliantly to repeat the victory of thirty years earlier. Sadly, it was not to be. But no one leaving the stadium that evening was disappointed.

Adrenaline and excitement had Donal in the highest spirits. The whole Thomond spectacle had been a great boost for him. We stayed in Limerick with my mother that night. For the first night in six weeks, Donal slept for the full nine hours. No cough. The following day we headed for Dublin and made our way to the Ronald McDonald House for another night of solid sleep. And no cough to be heard.

I was developing an ever greater appreciation for the way in which outside forces can enhance the body's curative powers. Donal had probably had the most exciting night of his life in Thomond Park and this had driven his adrenaline levels through the roof. It was the cure he needed for the cough that refused to go away. And he was also getting some well-earned sleep prior to starting his next dose of chemotherapy.

We were now heading towards the Advent and Christmas season. Jema's end-of-term exam results had improved significantly and we knew we were closer to achieving the kind of balance that everyone required. When my brother Tom organised two tickets for Donal to attend the Clermont v Munster Heineken Cup game, I was unable to take time off work, so I reluctantly handed over my ticket to Elma. She rang me after the match and spoke about Donal's determination as he swung his crutches towards the steps leading to the supporters' area, eager to discuss the result with the team that had befriended him. 'He was like a man on a mission,' she recalled.

Elma described the night in glowing terms and had obviously enjoyed it as much as Donal. A new Munster fan had been born, and we joked that it might not be so easy for me to hang on to my ticket for the next match! In the darkest of times, these outings kept our spirits up. We were able to put the future and the problems we faced to one side, even if only for a brief, but very welcome, interlude.

I'd kept my ties with the rugby club where I was helping to train the under–12s. At the start of the season I'd been unsure if this would be a good idea, but helping Jim, the trainer, was a respite from the constant worry about Donal. It also kept up a line of contact between Donal and his friends on the team and meant that during his stints in hospital, I could keep him abreast of everything that was going on back home.

At times Donal felt cut adrift from his peers. During the whole period he was receiving chemotherapy, he was highly susceptible to infection so, even when he was on his week off from treatment, visits to the house by his friends or cousins were often restricted. We were in the middle of the winter 'bug' season and if anyone had a cold or cough, they were advised to stay away. He was disappointed when visits had to be cancelled and also disliked being confined indoors for a lot of the time. For a boy who had never sat still in his life, this was difficult for him. He loved our family dog, Orla and had always exercised her regularly. Sadly, his cancer and the protection he needed from germs meant that he and Orla were not able to spend prolonged periods of time together. This was tough, not just for him but for Orla, who pined for her friend and was unable to understand why the familiar petting and face-licking had to stop.

The kindness of people who knew of his predicament continued to surprise and touch us. Members of Tralee RFC were anxious to do something for him. Earlier, when Donal had first been diagnosed with cancer, I'd been approached by someone from the club, with whom I'd worked closely to develop the youth section. He'd tentatively asked how we were fixed financially to deal with the expenses that lay ahead. I'd told him we were okay but, in truth, at the time we had no idea of the financial implications of Donal's illness. This man then informed me that a group of friends in the club were discussing our problem – and that if we needed help, we were not to hesitate to contact them. I was deeply moved by their concern and the sense that our community was closing around us in a supportive circle. I'd also experienced that same support from members of my own family of course, and their generosity helped cushion us when things became more difficult. Friends and family, in quiet ways, were showing how much they cared.

Now, with Christmas almost upon us, the members of the rugby club had organised a collection to buy a gift for Donal, and my friend there sought my advice as to what he needed. Someone suggested a laptop. This would allow Donal to keep in contact with his friends through Facebook. We had been reluctant to allow him and Jema unrestricted access to social media, but everything was different now. It would help Donal enormously to have that immediate link to his friends when he was away from home. Elma and I agreed that the club would buy Donal his laptop and we would buy Jema an exact replica for Christmas. This was done, and Donal was delighted with his gift. It made the distance from home seem a little less daunting. He quickly learned how to use the laptop to its full advantage and had instant access to all that was happening at home in his absence.

We tried to make the Christmas celebrations that year as happy and as holy as possible. Donal spent a lot of time thinking about his impending operation. This would be the final break with his old life. A new future awaited him and he, like us, had absolutely no idea what it held for him. But for the moment, we had some distractions from such sombre thoughts. When a Wii was introduced to the house as the family present, it was an immediate success. We'd lots of fun with Mario Racing and the various games we could play on screen: golf, bowling, tennis and boxing. Our muscles ached in the mornings, but it was a small price to pay for the enjoyment we shared together as a family.

The New Year passed off without incident and the clock ticked down inexorably to 8 January 2009, when Donal's operation would be performed.

Chapter Fifteen

On the day of Donal's operation we accompanied him to the theatre entrance. We watched as he was wheeled away, his own fears clutched tightly inside him. And we could do nothing but wait. His operation would take over four hours, and Margaret advised us to keep ourselves busy. We drove from Cappagh Hospital into the centre of the city, where we passed those agonising hours looking for an iPod docking station for Donal and adding to the Lego car collection he'd received from friends at Christmas.

He was two hours in theatre before we got the first report. The operation was going slower than expected but all was well. Two more hours dragged by. It must be over by now, we thought. Not so, Margaret told us, when we phoned. The diseased bone area had been removed and a cross-section sent to the lab in the Mater Hospital. This was to ensure that the complete tumour had been contained. There was still a long way to go. Another two hours passed. Calls from our families and friends assured us that prayers were being offered and candles were blazing across the world for Donal. I thought of Elma's brother Maurice in England and Fr Michael, my brother who ministers in Nigeria, and our relations in Australia, South Africa, Canada, the USA – also, all our business friends and the friendships we'd formed in so many different parts of the world. I imagined their candles forming a bonfire of hope and their prayers rising in a wave of positive healing energy to the heavens.

Margaret assured us once more that Donal's vital signs were good. The team had nearly finished assembling the prosthesis. Our emotions were stretched to the limit, the tension almost impossible to endure. If we saw another shop or café, we'd collapse. We simply had to get back to the hospital and sit it out. And so we waited and waited ...

We sat in the hospital canteen and tried to eat something. One of the anaesthetists who had been looking after Donal came into the canteen for his evening meal while we were there. We asked if the operation was finished. He shook his head. Two anaesthetists were looking after Donal, it seemed, while this doctor took a well-earned break. Nine-and-a-half hours after he went into surgery, we were finally called to see our son.

Donal was just coming around. Mr Dudeney asked him to wiggle his toes and move his foot, to check that the feeling was returning. He did so and we cried tears of relief that everything had gone according to plan. Later, we would appreciate the fact that Mr Dudeney and his assistant had spent nine-and-a-half hours in 'space suits', standing beside our son as they completed his surgery without a break.

Before the operation Donal had been very worried about the

number of stitches he would need on his leg. He was afraid it would look deformed and that he would never be able to wear shorts or swimming togs again. He'd expressed the same worry to Mr Dudeney, who had obviously listened to his patient more closely than even we anticipated. The eighteen-inch scar that stretched from Donal's mid-thigh to mid-calf had only one external stitch. The rest of the wound was held together by Steri-Strip sutures. The only scarring would be a pencil line that no one would notice except at very close quarters. Mr Dudeney and his team had taken about an hour longer than was necessary, to ensure that they got this result for Donal. About six such replacements are undertaken each year by Mr Dudeney, and he had practised at home three times on the eve of the operation to ensure that the prosthesis would be assembled correctly.

Donal would be in the intensive care unit for the next few days and Margaret was back on duty by 7 a.m. the following morning to check that all was going as planned. These professionals are my heroes. I've witnessed their dedication at close quarters, experienced their compassion and been influenced forever by their humanity.

Over the following days Elma and I shared our son's bedside vigil. One of us was there whenever he awoke, to reassure him all was well. On the day following his operation, Jema travelled to Dublin with her class to visit the Young Scientist Exhibition in the RDS. It was wonderful to have her close to us and we were able to stay together as a family for a couple of days. On one of her visits to the ward, she and I were asked to go outside while the nurses and Elma gave Donal a body wash. Donal's agonised screams as this function was performed were clearly audible to both of us. I could see the shock on my daughter's face, her desire to run from the hospital with her hands over her ears. I understood her reaction. I'd experienced the same helplessness myself on many occasions. We'd sheltered her from the worst effects of Donal's treatment but his raw screams gave her a sense of the enormity of what he was enduring.

To my surprise, on the Friday after the operation I got a call from Paul O'Connell to see how it had gone. This was just the perk Donal needed. Little miracles born from kindness gave him strength and, boy, did they work. We saw how it lifted his spirits whenever a text arrived from Paul, encouraging him to keep his chin up and make a speedy recovery.

Elma stayed in Cappagh with him for the three weeks following his operation, while I returned to work. I managed to give her an occasional break at the weekends. As Donal began his physiotherapy and learned to walk again, it was another tough period for him. The strain on his face told its own story but his determination shone through his pain.

Elma tells two particular stories about Donal at that time. The first involved a patient who had had a hip replacement before Donal had his knee operation. As she looked at him struggling to get to his feet each day, while she sat in her wheelchair, she commented to the physiotherapist that Donal Walsh was putting her to shame. 'After what he has been through, *yes* he is,' the physiotherapist replied. Whether or not this blunt approach had any effect on the patient in question is hard to know but the courage and determination of our son were clear.

The second story involved a small, lively older woman, who was doing her daily workouts with great vigour. One day she turned to Donal and said, 'You have youth on your side and I have wisdom on mine. Between the two of us, we'll get through this together.' We later discovered that she was from a famous Irish circus family. Her promise to Donal was that they both would run or cycle around the circus ring the next time the circus came to Tralee for the Festival of Kerry! Afterwards, I tried to get them together again but, unfortunately, I never managed to organise what would have been a most enjoyable reunion.

As if to reward Donal for his efforts, a most unexpected group of visitors arrived into his ward one afternoon. A friend of one of our neighbours, who worked with the Leinster branch of the Irish Rugby Football Union, had told some of the players there about Donal and his ordeals. He was amazed when the door opened that day, and Felipe Contepomi, Girvan Dempsey and Shane Jennings entered. They wanted to see how he was doing and wish him well. They even brought Ireland and Leinster gear as gifts to help cheer him up. He was so excited to see them that I began to wonder if this staunch Munster rugby supporter was going to switch sides! I knew the answer, of course. The rivalry between the Munster and Leinster rugby teams is as legendary as their respective fan bases, and Donal stayed steadfast in his loyalty. But that did not stop him being thrilled by this unexpected event, and he maintained contact with the Leinster players after that first visit. In fact, Shane became a close family friend who kept in regular touch to see how he was getting on.

After the operation and three weeks of physiotherapy, Donal was released from captivity and discharged from Cappagh Hospital. An ambulance blared its siren on the journey to Dublin Airport, where all was in readiness to lift him onto the Ryanair flight to Kerry. I know that Ryanair are often in the news for all the wrong reasons but on this occasion, the staff bent over backwards to ensure that our son was as comfortable as possible. They even gave him three seats on the plane at no extra cost to us. When he and Elma arrived at Kerry Airport, it took three flight crew and ground staff to lift him from the plane. Again, this was done with skill and gentleness.

A new chapter was beginning for us all now.

Chapter Sixteen
Donal's Story

My operation in January was the toughest thing I have ever had to do. I was weak. I lost 23 kilograms and I was still sick. I didn't realise how tough it was going to be, until I woke up. It was nine-and-a-half hours long. I woke up with two tubes on my leg, an epidural, six cannulas and a catheter.

After two nights in intensive care, I was moved to the children's ward. After four days of just lying down, I eventually ate something. Then the head nurse came in early and spoke with my mom. They thought I was asleep. She said she was going to remove the tubes and the less I knew, the better. I wish I was asleep. She asked could she look at my back, where the epidural was. I told her I knew what was happening. She pulled it out quickly, I felt it slither out and then a sharp pain pierced my spine. I screamed. I begged her to go slow for the drainage tubes. But she said it would be easier if it was quick. One went and I felt it tear out. Straight away she took the second one and it felt as bad as the first one. There was blood on the curtains from the speed they came out at.

'Now for the catheter.' I was petrified at this stage. She began to disconnect it and then I felt a massive balloon pop in my bladder. And then I asked how would the balloon come out. 'Like this,' she said, and I could see her dragging it as it burned me.

'That wasn't too bad, was it?' she attempted to explain. She had dealt with patients like me for years and knew about the pain we had to suffer, and she was going to make sure I went through it for good reasons, not bad. She tried to make it hurt as little as she possibly could.

The pain I felt that day was the worst I ever encountered and it wasn't over. I had three weeks of rehabilitation left because I had to learn how to walk again. And it started that day.

My physiotherapist came around at 11 a.m. and I sat out for the first time. She said, 'We might get you down to the gym tomorrow.'

I said, 'Tomorrow? Can we not start today?' She was shocked but happy. I was in the gym by 3 p.m.

In the gym there were two bars that were waist-high and about ten metres long. I looked at them and asked, 'Will I be doing them?'

She said, 'Yeah, about three times today.'

I said to myself I was doing them six times. I managed five and I was disappointed.

The next day I did them eight times. While I was in the gym, the other physiotherapists would tell patients how I had four times more metal in my leg than anyone else in the hospital, that I didn't move for four days and I'm three weeks ahead of where I should be for walking.

When I was in there, all I cared about was getting out – if that meant going through all that pain, I would do it. I still do. If I want something, I go get it. I don't wait around for something to happen. I make it happen.

They said I'd be off crutches in six months. I went for a six-week check-up and gave my crutches back.

Chapter Seventeen

The next few weeks flew by, as Donal became more mobile each day. He pushed himself as far as he could and we encouraged him every step of the way, literally. He dreaded the thought of having to suffer further chemotherapy but was resigned to the fact that it had to be done.

Back in Crumlin Hospital, Elma was given the news we longed to hear. Donal had a 100 per cent cure on his cancer. A delighted Michael Capra delivered this information. Elma saw the same delight and relief reflected on the faces of his entire medical team. When she rang me with the results, I felt as if something menacing and terrifying had lifted from my shoulders. I could breathe freely again. My heart could stop racing to the questions – what if? What if all this doesn't work? What then? I was never able to think beyond that point.

The only snag – and it was a big one – was that Donal still had to complete another six months of chemotherapy. 'But why?' he argued strenuously with us. 'The tumour's gone, so I shouldn't need any more chemo. You've no idea what it's like. You can't make me have it.'

He wanted to go home, back to school, back to his friends, back to normality. Six months of vomiting and reacting from an infusion of poison seemed like an eternity. We tried to placate him and not add to his fears, by revealing the possibility of a secondary cancer returning if he did not complete the last part of his treatment. Eventually, we told him to discuss his objections with his oncologist. Michael Capra was always willing to listen to his worries and answer any questions. But when he sat down with Donal to have this discussion, our son was uncharacteristically silent.

After Michael left the ward, we asked Donal where all his questions had gone.

He shrugged, defeated. 'All he would tell is the same stuff you've been saying for the last week. It has to be done.'

I guess, subconsciously, he realised there was no way out. He knew that his medical team – whether they were in Crumlin or Cappagh or Kerry General – had one thing in common. They wanted nothing less than his complete recovery as quickly as possible. He couldn't demand any more than that and they, in return, had to expect the same resolve from him.

On Valentine's Day 2009, I arrived in Crumlin to take over from Elma. Not much chance of flowers and hearts on this occasion. Donal was back in the horrors of chemotherapy and we were working hard at keeping everything together. Brenda Donohue from the Derek Mooney afternoon show was visiting the Ronald McDonald House with the singer, Jack L. He performed an outstanding concert that evening and Brenda had an opportunity to see at first hand the work the Ronald

McDonald House did. I was asked, along with some other parents, to give an interview about the house. It was broadcast the following afternoon. This brought an immediate response from friends with whom we'd lost touch over the years. They were shocked when they heard what Donal was going through but, thankfully, in the midst of all this suffering, there were organised events that lifted him, and others like him, out of the constant hospital routine.

One of those highlights was the Meteor Awards in the RDS, held on St Patrick's Day that year. A group of young patients were invited to attend and all were looking forward to the occasion. But that excitement was mixed with apprehension, as none of them knew until the last minute if they would be able to go. Any difficulty with their bloods, any sniffles or coughs, or a bout of vomiting could mean they would have to stay behind. Anxiety was rife throughout St John's Ward, as they waited for their blood tests to come back from the lab.

A VIP bus arrived and carried them away. They stopped off on the way to eat at Eddie Rocket's. Donal was attending his first real concert gig without his parents. Admittedly, a full crew of medical personnel accompanied them but they remained discreetly alert and observant without intruding on the young people's enjoyment.

Such occasions lifted their mood for days afterwards but they could never take them for granted. When the Irish Navy invited a group out to see one of their ships, Donal and I went along. We were excited by the idea of exploring the interior of the ship, but five minutes after going aboard we received the dreaded call. Donal had to return to the ward immediately for a treatment. He was extremely disappointed but that was the reality of hospital life.

Jema was too big-hearted to resent the special attention Donal was receiving but, if possible, we tried to involve her in these treats – sometimes with hilarious results. On one occasion when Donal was in the throes of his post-operative therapy, he and a group of patients, past and present, from St John's Ward were invited to attend the U2 summer concert in Croke Park. This proved to be a memorable occasion, with The Edge hosting the patients in a private suite before the concert began.

In order to ensure there was no favouritism, we bought Jema and her friend Christina tickets for the gig. She was excited at the idea of attending her first concert without parental supervision and, for once, was on an equal footing with her competitive brother. But as I drove her and Christina towards Croke Park, a motorcycle garda escort swerved towards us on their distinctive motorbikes. They roared past all the cars that were snarled in traffic, including ours, and proceeded inwards towards Croke Park. They were in fact escorting a special bus filled with concert goers from Crumlin Hospital to the U2 concert – and Donal was sitting grandly among them!

The concert that followed was an unforgettable experience for both of them. Having seen U2 in Rome in 1987 when I was a student, I was happy to wait for Donal and Jema in a hotel across the road. From my vantage point I could hear the concert clearly. What the decibel levels inside the stadium were like, I can only imagine.

Chapter Eighteen
Donal's Story

I still had six months of chemo. Along with removing my knee, it would mean that the cancer wouldn't come back, and I was willing to do that. But the chemo was hitting me hard. I might faint instead of sleep and I was losing weight fast. On 10 March, I reached my lowest weight, weighing only four-and-a-half stone. I hadn't eaten for twenty-eight days. My mom brought me to Kerry General Hospital. From there, they brought me to Crumlin. I was given a nasogastric tube and I was fed through that. It was a tube that went through my nose and ran all the way down to my stomach. I had failed myself and I was devastated. In the end, it turned out that the tube was a good thing. It gave me energy and I even began to eat a little again.

Chapter Nineteen

In the early stages of Donal's illness, he'd received a visit from a representative of the Make-A-Wish Foundation. The idea behind Make-A-Wish is that seriously sick children have the opportunity to wish for that one special thing they'd like. It could be a desire to meet with a special person or to visit some place they've always wanted to see. Donal thought long and hard about what his wish would be. He had met all his heroes, who were mainly the Munster team, and, more latterly, the Leinster players. As far as he was concerned, there was no particular place he wanted to visit. He'd spent enough time travelling from Kerry to Dublin and back again. Now, all he wanted was to stay close to home.

'What I really want is something physical to remember the way my life has changed,' he told us. We knew he was thinking about the dreams he once had of playing rugby for Munster, or maybe football for Kerry – or just being able to play for his own satisfaction. 'If my wish can be granted, I'd like to have a proper drum shed that can also be used as a den by me and

Jema and all our friends.' The 'Girls Out' decree had ceased to be an issue.

As I mentioned earlier, when Donal took up drumming lessons, we'd kitted him out with a drum set and a shed to practise in. The shed was small – 8 foot by 6 foot – but he'd practised regularly and become quite a good drummer. Now he wanted to play again, but in more spacious surroundings. He was ready with his request when the Make-A-Wish Foundation came calling again. We were conscious of the cost involved, and advised the Foundation that if his wish exceeded the budget, we would look at paying the balance. We were quickly assured that this was not an issue and that they would get working on the project immediately.

Donal's illness had opened the door into a new world where charity is in abundance and the goodwill of strangers is humbling to witness. He was enduring his post-operative chemo, when work began on making his wish come true. We were astonished and delighted by the plans that were drawn up for the shed. At 25 foot by 25 foot, it would cover a sizable portion of our garden and was like building an extra room to the house. We planned to surprise him when he came home for a break from his chemo, so timing was of the essence. Many people became involved, all working frantically to meet the deadline.

The Irish Cabin Company took up residence in our garden for a week. They organised the electrics, the carpet and sofas for the den. The garden was looking the worse for wear after the erection of the shed, but the staff from Ballyseedy Garden Centre arrived one day. without prior announcement, to renew and repair it. The way everyone worked together was a lesson in cooperation and generosity. Debbie and Dee from Make-A-Wish managed the time very well and kept us on our toes as the date for Donal's arrival home drew closer.

When all was ready, they asked us to organise that his friends from his football and rugby clubs would be part of the welcoming group. The Make-A-Wish shed was able to hold about fifty young people, and they filled it to capacity. The excitement grew, as some of the footballers from the Kerry team – namely Tommy Walsh, David Moran and Micheál Quirke – also came along for the opening ceremony. Anticipation was high, as everyone waited in silence for the unsuspecting Donal to appear.

When the car pulled into the driveway, Donal was thrilled as he noticed the new addition to the garden. The drum shed exceeded all his expectations. When he entered and saw everyone waiting to welcome him home, he was astonished and elated. Even though he was exhausted from the treatment, he stayed there partying until late that evening.

What I call the 'Positive Curing Care' continued throughout Donal's illness. When he was recovering from his operation, for example, he had been invited to Limerick to meet the Irish rugby squad at their hotel before an international. When we arrived, we were met by his mates from both Munster and Leinster. The Leinster guys tried to adopt him, but there was no way the Munster lads were letting him go. It was fun to watch how both camps fussed over him. Declan Kidney, the then Irish coach, talked about rugby for fifteen minutes to this bald young boy on crutches with a tube out of his nose. Only at the end of the conversation did Declan (pretending not to know) ask, 'Are you under treatment for something or what?'

'Bone cancer,' Donal replied and filled him in on the details of his treatment.

Declan leaned in towards him and said, 'My mother and brother had cancer too and they both came out the other end. And you will too. So keep fighting!'

I could see the visible effect this had on Donal. It renewed his resolve to do as Declan advised, and keep fighting.

But it was hard to constantly keep our spirits up.

In the hospital we were surrounded by other parents, who were facing the same fears and anxieties, yet we all had to try to remain positive for the sake of our sick children. This became extremely difficult when one of the young patients didn't make it, and word filtered throughout the hospital. It was particularly devastating when this happened in St John's. Donal would go quiet when such tragedies occurred and emerge more determined than ever to survive. My pride in him reached new levels as I witnessed his resolve, but how I wished there had been another reason – any other reason – for the swelling of my heart as he pulled the beanie cap over his shorn head to welcome his visitors.

We also heard of marvellous occurrences. They kept us going, these stories of cures that verged on the miraculous. While Donal was receiving his chemo, we heard about the birth of a premature baby to a member of our extended family. At twenty-two weeks, this tiny mite weighed only one pound. Her mother could fit her own wedding ring up beyond her child's miniscule elbow. Her chances of survival were so limited that we received photos of her shortly after her birth. To add to her problems, she needed open heart surgery when she was only a few weeks old. This operation was performed in Crumlin, so, while Donal was in St John's, his little cousin spent a day in theatre. How could she possibly survive such serious surgery, we wondered. All we could do was pray. Today she is happily running around, the embodiment of a perfect living angel.

On good days, Donal was very good. On the bad days, he was allowed to have some self-pity. This could drag us down with him however, so we tried to discourage him from giving way to such feelings. We talked about taking a family walk on the beach when he was discharged ... we would leave our footprints in the sand. His prosthesis would make no difference. His footprints would be as firm and strong as before.

He had fought a good fight, but he was about to make contact with someone whose own battle against almost impossible odds would have an inspirational effect on him.

Chapter Twenty
Donal's Story

I had a friend, Stuart Mangan. He said he wasn't brave because he didn't have a choice. He didn't have a choice to be paralysed, but he chose to live every day of his life with a smile on his face and even though he knew he didn't have long to live, he spent the time he had designing technology for people who would end up like him. That, to me, is brave and inspirational.

Chapter Twenty-One

I sometimes wonder if God picks our friends, or picks a special one who will make a lasting impression on us. For Donal, this was Stuart Mangan. I heard his name for the first time when his aunt, Sheila Sugrue, approached Tralee RFC, asking if we would organise a charity quiz night to support the Stuart Mangan fundraising campaign. Stuart, who was from Cork but living in London, had been a keen and talented young rugby player. He had everything going for him: a successful career, a wonderful family, good friends and a loving relationship. Then, in April 2008, at the age of twenty-four, he suffered a catastrophic accident on the rugby pitch. It was a C2 fracture, that damaged the nerves in his body and left him paralysed from his neck down.

Shortly after meeting Sheila, Paul O'Connell appeared on *The Late Late Show* and made the same appeal for the Stuart Mangan campaign. Donal, hearing Paul's request, wanted to know what had happened to Stuart, how the accident had occurred and what limitations it had placed on his future. He began to research this remarkable young man on the internet. The more he discovered about him, the more inspired he was by Stuart's determination to live his life as fully as possible. Stuart was working with researchers in an effort to achieve technological advancements in the care of paralysed people. The Stuart Mangan Assisted Research Technology team had improved his speech with the assistance of a computer, and he planned to work on a microphone that would allow him to project and control his speech volume. Stuart had been an expert horseman, and hoped to design a special brace so that he could ride again. Amazingly, he was also considering the possibilities of skydiving with the help of a fellow skydiver and a zip line.

One evening Donal came to me with an idea. 'You know the way I get lots of presents because I'm sick?' he said. 'What if I bought a Munster jersey and asked Paul to get the lads to sign it. I could give it to Stuart's family to auction for his fund.' I thought this was an excellent idea and we immediately contacted the fundraisers through their website. They got in touch shortly afterwards and informed us that the idea had been passed on to Stuart's family, who would be in contact with us soon.

Two days later I received a call from Stuart's brother, Keith. He said the family really appreciated the efforts Donal was making to help them, despite his own condition. We spoke about our own personal situations and how tragedy can strike so suddenly and with such devastating results. Buoyed up by the encouragement of the Mangan family, Donal contacted his rugby friends, who were more than happy to oblige. He and Stuart then began to email each other. Donal was still undergoing his chemo at the time, and he took great heart from the simple emails of encouragement he received back from Stuart. Both had seen their lives change radically and could empathise with each other's very different experiences. Stuart was showing so much determination to live as fully as possible, even though he needed a ventilator to breathe and twenty-four-hour care. This knowledge would have a profound effect on Donal, whose treatment was coming to a conclusion.

Time dragged. Now that he knew the end was in sight, our son was becoming increasingly restless. The Lions tour of South Africa began around the same time. Nine Munster, five Leinster and one Ulster player were selected as part of the Lions squad, and watching the matches on television kept Donal occupied. Texts would arrive from Paul, who was captaining the squad. We were touched and amazed that he remembered Donal between those hectic matches, and took the time to let him know he cared.

This terrible treatment, that had wrecked our lives for the better part of nine months, was almost over. Recovery from cancer is mental as well as physical. For almost a year Donal had been in a pain-filled bubble, with just occasional flashes of enjoyment and excitement. His positive attitude, even when things were at their worst, had endeared him to many, including the celebrities he met. But everything we did had been focused on him. Now, suddenly, he had to adjust and become an ordinary boy again. Soon he would leave the staff he had grown to love in Crumlin, and the patients he had befriended. He would also have to say goodbye to the medical team in Cashel Children's

Ward in Kerry General, who had been his local back-up team. The nurses were experts when it came to cajoling and coaxing him through his many blood tests, the changing of his dressings and any emergencies that might occur when he was at home. What had been a torturous routine had become familiar to him and, in ways, was by now a regular part of his life.

Sadly and shockingly, in August 2009, Stuart lost his fight for life – just as it was confirmed that our son had won his battle. Donal's hair was beginning to grow again and he was putting on weight when he attended Stuart's funeral. Although he was still weak from his treatment and needed support throughout the ceremony, he would not have missed the opportunity to say goodbye to someone who'd lifted his spirits and made him believe in the power of mind over matter.

Stuart's funeral must have been one of the biggest Cork had ever seen. This was our first direct encounter with his family and I felt quite emotional towards the end of the ceremony, when a dove was released. As the bird rose gracefully into the air, I thought of Stuart looking down on us as he began his journey towards the light.

After Stuart's passing we were at a loss to know what to do with the framed, signed and valued Munster jersey. Donal decided it should still go to Stuart's family. A few weeks after the funeral we visited Sheila, Stuart's aunt. We presented the jersey to her, with the request that when a suitable opportunity arose, it could be auctioned off to raise funds in Stuart's memory. The proceeds could be used to help others in a similar situation.

DONAL'S MOUNTAIN

In July 2009, Donal had his Hickman line removed. Another step towards normality was achieved. He was now thirteen years old and anxious to catch up on the lost year of his life. A visit to Barretstown camp was planned. Barretstown, founded by the late actor, Paul Newman, is located in County Kildare and modelled on Newman's Hole in the Wall Gang Camp in Connecticut, USA which was opened in 1988 as a place where children coping with serious illnesses could have a special hideout where they could simply be kids. Barretstown, situated in a splendid castle near Ballymore Eustace, was opened in 1994. Children from Ireland, Britain and throughout Europe visit the camp to have fun together but, just as importantly, to be helped to regain their confidence and self-esteem, which can be affected through cancer and other serious illnesses. Donal had been looking forward to the experience for weeks. We, too, hoped for the opportunity for a short respite from the constant strain of looking after our seriously ill son. Virtually no contact would be allowed between us for a ten-day period, unless there was a problem with Donal's health.

However, Barretstown was not meant to be, at least not on that occasion. Although Donal was gaining weight, his appetite was poor. For a boy who loved his food, this was serious. After a day trip to Dingle, where he was unable to eat a half bowl of soup and a few chips, we knew we were in trouble. We became increasingly worried when we noticed his stomach was retaining fluid. He'd developed a stomach infection and Elma travelled with him to Dublin by emergency ambulance. Once again, we were in the eye of the storm. I was at home waiting for the call, terrified that all our hopes and dreams were about to be dashed once again. This was serious, a race against time, but we still had no idea what was causing the problem. Donal was too sick to be dismayed by this new setback. Once again he was admitted to St John's Ward and, once again, we waited in dread for test results. Lungs, heart, kidney, liver, bloods: everything that could be causing this weight gain was examined. Some scarring, not unlike sclerosis, was discovered on his liver and he spent the next fortnight having the fluid drained from his system. We would later discover that, if this problem had been ignored any longer, he would have had a heart attack. Once again, we were aware that there was no room for complacency. The fragile thread that kept Donal with us could so easily be snapped.

He made it to Barretstown for the Open Day, however, during that time and Elma took him there in a wheelchair. His medical team in Crumlin were anxious to see if he was stable enough to return to Kerry, and this was a half-way test. He spent the night with his mother in a hotel, then headed for Barretstown the following day. The photographs taken at that time show him looking gaunt, stubble-haired and with the sunken eyes of a concentration camp victim, his weight down to six stone. But Barretstown was still a memorable visit. A number of sports stars – including Munster rugby player Donncha O'Callaghan, Cork hurler Seán Óg Ó hAilpín and 'Jayo', the famous Jason Sherlock, former Dublin Gaelic footballer and League of Ireland soccer player – had turned up to meet and mingle with the children. As soon as Elma arrived, Donncha

O'Callaghan grabbed Donal's wheelchair and took him for a walk around the grounds of Barretstown. They talked about rugby and, although Donal might not have been in the best of spirits, this encounter perked him up no end. I've built up a huge respect for these busy professional sportsmen, who give up their time so willingly to visit sick children in hospital. I've seen at first hand the impact they have and how the memories of those visits stay with the children long after they leave. Our son could not have wished for a more positive inspiration to help him on the occasions when he was at his lowest ebb.

Donal returned home from that hospital stay with even more determination to get back to full health. The treats and presents slowed down, as did the round-the-clock attention he'd become used to receiving. We all had to adjust, and that included myself and Elma. We could not burden him with our anxieties if he coughed or blew his nose.

Our son's life was now all about targets, ones he set for himself, or ones we or his medical team devised for him. Just as, after his operation in January, he'd determined to do without his crutches as quickly as possible – and managed to do so, in record time, much to the surprise and even shock of those around him – now he set himself new goals and achieved each of them in turn. Now he wanted to start cycling. Getting back on his bike would give him independence as well as the exercise he needed for his mobility. I had to hold the saddle and follow him up and down the road until there was no danger of him taking a tumble. We knew the fragility of the new knee and what damage he could do if he lost his balance.

Unthinkable!

Donal's bike gave him the freedom to cycle at the same pace as his friends. Equality was his real motivation, and slowly this was coming back to him. After a few days of holding the saddle, I eventually let go, and he was off. The distance was not very long but sufficient to increase his confidence.

A new school year would begin again in September. He would have to repeat First Year, as he had only spent three days in CBS The Green before that terrifying call from Fionán, which had set the whole train of events in motion. Now he was planning to be able to cycle to school as fast as any of his friends and setting himself another target. We agreed that if he was able to cycle to the local shop and back on his own, we would buy him a new bike. It only took two weeks for him to meet this challenge and we took great pride in his achievement when we presented him with his reward.

Donal's hair was growing back, his weight improving, the colour returning to his cheeks. The positive, curative approach that Elma and I had adopted from the beginning was reflected in his own attitude. He used whatever sources he could find to help him make a full recovery. He became friends with a Reiki healer, whom he trusted completely. She was able to reassure him that the cancer had been removed from his bones and to encourage him to work at building back the energy that had been so depleted by the chemotherapy.

On the first morning of term we discovered that his uniform, which had been a perfect fit the previous year, was hanging on him. I was immediately sent out to buy him a new pair of trousers. Not easy in Tralee at 8 o'clock in the morning. I eventually managed to find a pair in a local supermarket. Wrong colour but right size, and they would see him through his first day back at school.

But cycling to school would have to wait until he was stronger. Initially, he was too weak to manage his schoolbag and Elma had to carry it to his locker for him. She would call again in the evening to pick it up. I'm sure Donal was mortified by this dependence on us, but he endured it until he had enough strength to manage by himself. Within a few weeks he was able to cope on his own and we had to stand back and allow him that freedom.

Returning to school challenged him mentally and physically, and often exhausted him. He was academically strong in all subjects, especially Science, Woodwork and Technical Drawing. The school, with its strong sporting record, was a stark reminder however that things had changed forever for Donal. Yet his gruelling illness had not changed his competitive personality. If anything, that competitive streak had been strengthened by the experience. He went to incredible lengths to become fit again and worked out regularly with weights in the gym and in his den, to build back his strength. He returned to the 'Naries' to train with his friends, although he knew he would never again be picked for the team or be able for the demands a match would place on his prosthetic knee. To come to terms with this reality was tough, but he remained positive and dealt with the limitations that had been placed on him. He fell once during a training session and came down hard on his knee. I saw the shocked pain on his face and had to prevent myself from rushing forward to help him up. I held back, knowing he would never forgive me if I singled him out. He picked himself up, as I'd known he would do, and continued training. He was reclaiming his life and my position was on the sideline. I suspect he often fell during those early months, but I never heard a word about it from him. He refused to be considered sick or different, someone to be cosseted or, worst of all, to be pitied. I ached for him as I watched his struggle but I also believed it would be his salvation. Cancer had matured him beyond his years and the 'why me?' question was never brought up for discussion.

Donal was enjoying First Year, where he made many new friends, among them Cormac Coffey, James O'Connor and Hugh Stuart. Another close friend was John Kelly, whom he knew from rugby, and the five boys developed a close, lasting friendship. One evening I heard a familiar sound coming from the den. Donal was playing the drums. Soon the den became a regular hang-out spot for him and his friends. They scrawled their signatures on the walls, where Donal had stencilled the mottos: *Leave no stone unturned*, *Leave your fears behind* and *Each day is a gift. It's not a given right.*

Another Christmas was upon us. A happier one this year. We had a visit from Stuart Mangan's parents, who came to our home to thank Donal for his generous gesture and the concern he had shown for Stuart. Even though our two sons had had such a brief encounter, and were never to meet, they helped each other in their own different ways. Stuart had been a tremendous source of inspiration for Donal. I'd like to believe his parents saw in Donal a kindred spirit of their own beloved son. We were deeply touched that they chose to visit us on that first Christmas after Stuart's passing, to say thank you to our own son, who was now on the road to recovery.

Chapter Twenty-Two

My own life had also changed in a way I'd never envisaged. At the end of September 2008, the announcement of a Government bank guarantee officially signalled that the boom was over. It seemed to happen almost overnight and the effect was immediate. An emergency budget was introduced, and there were dire government warnings of worse to come. This collapse occurred around the same time as Donal was beginning his first bout of chemotherapy. It was merely a backdrop to our lives at this point and hardly registered, as we tried to come to terms with the shock of our son's illness. As property prices collapsed, bank scandals unfolded and the dire predictions of economists filled the airwaves, we were more concerned with holding our family together and working out schedules to ensure we could be with our son at all times. But the domino effect of recession was soon hard to ignore, as companies folded, unemployment figures rose and young people emigrated.

'We are where we are', was an overused and much-hated political cliché of that time. What was it supposed to mean?

Unfortunately, I, and others like me, soon knew exactly where we were. Unemployed. One devastating knock in life does not necessarily shield you from a second one, as I discovered to my cost.

The hotel sector was severely affected by the recession and in April 2009, when Donal was still going through his chemotherapy, I lost my job and became an unemployment statistic like so many others. Being a statistic was difficult. It took time to adjust. I no longer had a clearly defined role as a provider to my family. That hurt more than I believed possible. I could have fallen into depression and, perhaps, that would have happened if Donal's illness and my experience in St John's Ward had not put everything else in perspective.

I needed to keep myself busy when I was at home on my own. In the mornings, after checking out the slimmed-down job vacancy columns, I'd go for a long walk or head to the rugby club, where there was always work to be done. I also made jams and chutneys. I'm inventive when it comes to experimenting with new recipes, and enjoy the mixing and stirring, the tasting for the perfect flavour, the bottling and labelling. I made enough to sell as a fundraiser, to buy new jerseys for the club. But this was a hobby and I needed a full-time job.

An opportunity came to work with two close friends. We set up a company – Six Nations Tours – to run youth rugby tours and events. This has been surprisingly successful, and I was able to bring together my coaching expertise, my background in communication management and my experience as a fixture coordinator. Being involved in this new venture was a welcome development at a time of crisis and I remained with the business until an opportunity came at a later date to return to work in the hotel industry.

As Donal continued to recover his full strength, we planned fundraising events together. No one who has had experience of Crumlin Hospital, especially St John's Ward, can remain unaffected by the work carried out there under such overcrowded conditions.

Donal had left St John's Ward filled with fundraising zeal. Although he was anxious to return to his old life, he was unable to shake off the knowledge that other young teens in St John's Ward were suffering from the same destructive disease. I was not surprised by his concern. Throughout his childhood I'd seen instances of his generosity. He'd think nothing of sharing treats or pocket money with friends or cousins and, when he was well enough during his time in hospital, he was one of the first to welcome a new patient and show them the ropes. But this was different. This was a 'cause'.

'They were looking to renovate the ward for the first time since the seventies, so I had to help,' he would later write in his account of his journey through cancer. 'They looked after me and I promised myself that I was going to do everything I could to look after them.'

He and I discussed how to fundraise for Crumlin Hospital. Ideas were put forward and rejected, analysed and found wanting for various reasons. Eventually we came up with the idea of 'Caints and Angels'. Yes, I know the word is 'Saints', but we looked at the crescent-shaped scar that, universally, is the mark of a cancer patient, the scar left from the Hickman or so-called 'Freddie' line. We decided that the letter 'c' should denote the cresent shape of this very symbolic scar, – hence 'Saints' would become 'Caints'. Donal envisaged an award ceremony led by the Irish President for the Caints – those who worked in Crumlin Hospital and treated their child patients with such compassionate care. As for the Angels, they needed no introduction. Donal had been one of them and, if fundraising could make a difference to their surroundings, then that was what he would do.

We came up with a novel idea of selling this crescent-shaped symbol through the schools of Ireland. We worked out the cost of setting up the Caints and Angels fund and creating a website to promote it. Unfortunately, we were dissuaded from this project on the advice of a businessman, who felt we were taking on too much and did not believe the schools would support it. We listened to this advice and dropped the idea. There are plans now to revive this fund in Donal's name, and I've no doubt it will be supported by every student in the country.

As his health continued to improve, Donal organised a number of fundraising events with friends and collected about €10,000 for St John's Ward. One of the first fundraisers was a fashion show, organised by his friend Cassie, who runs Cassie Leen's School of Dance in Tralee. She was one of his earliest babysitters and he became an enthusiastic follower of her dance troupe. This event raised €7,000. Andrew Grey, another friend and a pupil in Glenstal Abbey, raised around €1,000 by organising a recital, and a head shave among the students. This was just the beginning of the fundraising endeavours initiated by Donal, and he would later go on to increase these early sums raised many times over.

We also planned a special 'bed push' walk from the Aviva Stadium in Dublin to Thomond Park in Limerick in aid of Crumlin Hospital. We thought the Six Nations match between Ireland and France, due to take place in mid-February 2011, would provide the ideal opportunity. We plotted our route across the country and planned to stay with various rugby clubs along the way. It was an ambitious undertaking and Donal couldn't wait to get moving on it. The bed push would receive much-needed publicity for the planned refurbishment of Crumlin Hospital. For years, doctors, parents and patients had cried out for a national children's hospital. It should have been built during the boom years, when many millions were spent on extravagant projects like the controversial e-voting machines, the PPARS system and the abandoned 'Bertie Bowl' stadium. But, somehow, through all those years of extravagant spending, not a sod was turned on this desperately needed facility.

A site on the grounds of the Mater Hospital, in one of Dublin's busiest traffic areas, had been chosen but that would later be abandoned when planning permission was refused. Meanwhile, in a dedicated hospital like Crumlin, rooms that had originally been built to accommodate one family now had to be shared with a second family, and living conditions were becoming increasingly cramped. Something needed to be done in the immediate term.

Donal's first-hand experience of St John's had left him with a very clear idea of what was needed to improve the cancer ward. He had great affection for the nurses and doctors, but their compassion could not alter the fact that pre-teen and teenage patients were considered 'the forgotten tribe'. The décor of the wards and indeed most areas of the hospital was Disney-themed and thus more suitable for children under twelve. Young teens battling cancer are forced to grow up quickly. They are faced with grim, life-changing decisions, terrifying possibilities, and are probably more mature than many adults. As far as Donal was concerned, they needed care facilities better suited to their needs and tastes – especially a 'chill-out' area like his den, where they could congregate in private. Because patients were now sharing a room, young pre-teens and teenagers could end up with only a thin curtain between them and a seriously ill baby, along with the child's frantic parents. Donal had a particularly distressing memory of such an experience, and it had occurred just as his own treatment was ending.

Chapter Twenty-Three
Donal's Story

There were worse days. On the day of my last chemo, my parents went for lunch and I was alone. I was trying to sleep, but there was a baby next to me who was crying. Then he stopped, I heard a chair move suddenly and his mother began screaming. The crash alarm went off and the crash cart was brought in. At this stage his mother was shouting at him. The nurses were shouting at each other. I was praying. He didn't make it. My parents weren't allowed in the room for an hour. I was scared, and I don't know why, but I was angry. That day was one of the worst days of my life. To witness a child die, and his parents break down. I don't like to talk about it, because I still get scared and angry thinking about it.

Chapter Twenty-Four

Donal began to accompany me to the rugby training sessions. Only a year previously, his strength and height had dominated his team. It was too painful to think back to those very recent times though, and we both set our minds to the future. He began to assist me in setting up the equipment and I was relieved to see him integrate back into the club. Soon he was working with me as my assistant coach, but it was tough for him to stand on the sidelines watching the matches. He was single-minded about getting back into action and he began to carry out his own exercises regime on the side of the pitch while the others were playing.

A unique opportunity came his way when Eddie Barnes, the Head Coach at Tralee RFC, took him under his wing. Eddie discussed the physio programme Donal had done in Cappagh Hospital. It was tough and intensive, and Donal had learned a lot from it. Eddie advised him to use that knowledge to build up the whole squad's fitness levels. For Donal, this was a new way of thinking. What he had seen as a negative ordeal could now be used in a positive way. Initially, I was worried in case he damaged his prosthetic knee while demonstrating the exercises to the boys, but all the work he'd done to get himself fit paid off.

I began to understand the psychology behind Eddie's decision when I noticed the effect Donal's presence had on the squad. They knew what he had endured. He had had to work so hard at getting back on his feet and – literally – learning to walk again, that the players had a deep respect for him. 'Anything he asks of us is nothing that he has not already asked of himself,' was how one of the squad put it to me.

To be known as a fitness trainer, and not a cancer victim, gave Donal the status he badly needed. Even I was surprised at the energy and motivation this fourteen-year-old boy brought to the squad. When he asked them to do twenty press-ups, he got twenty press-ups. A mistake by any one player meant they all had to start again. Each time they had to restart, they were annoyed – not at Donal, but at the player who wasn't putting his heart and soul into the training session. Like everything else he did, Donal gave it 100 per cent commitment.

We had our differences of opinion. It was an unusual situation – to have an assistant coach who was the same age as his squad, especially one who was beginning to have an equal say in how the fitness regime was implemented. We were both stubborn and liked to have our own way. Donal was not behind the door in expressing his view and I, as squad manager, sometimes had to pull rank when we disagreed over the formation of the team. This caused some tension between us. But I could live with that.

These arguments, however heated, were quickly forgotten. They were proof that Donal's confidence was growing as the memories of St John's Ward faded into the background of our lives. The fact that he had the energy to argue his point of view and challenge my opinions proved he was well on the road to a full recovery. But nevertheless, we had a team to run. Donal had to appreciate the boundaries between me being his father, his friend and the team manager.

Tralee RFC was very supportive, and Donal was included in all the Munster Branch coach training courses, even though he was too young to attain any qualifications. He was given responsibilities beyond his years and his qualifications were unofficially recognised by the club. While he always had an adult coach by his side, for insurance reasons, all the coaches were impressed by his training tactics and determination.

After a year working with Eddie and myself, Donal left us to train the Under-13 squad. The traditional bellicose shouting and whistling that many Irish coaches use to control a band of teenagers was not Donal's way. He meticulously researched and planned each training session. He documented what had been achieved and what he hoped to achieve further down the line. Before starting each session, he advised the players on what he expected them to do, and he asked them for their comments when it was over.

On Donal's first night in his new position, Des Healy, his English teacher and a coach for one of the squads, handed him a whistle to control the boys. Donal returned this to him on his second night. The players respected their new coach and a whistle wasn't necessary. He never raised his voice, never shouted at a player and never told a team member that what he had done was wrong. Instead of this, when someone didn't do what was expected of him, Donal took him aside and suggested a different approach. I often thought that his quiet approach was more effective and got more results than my own shouting may have achieved, and I watched, fascinated, as his self-assurance developed. I knew, as did the other coaches, that we had someone special on our hands.

His relationship with Paul O'Connell continued. Donal texted him regularly. After each Munster match, for example, he would express his opinion on the game and how it could have been improved. After a particularly gruelling defeat for Munster, Donal had texted some positive comments to Paul, who later confessed to my brother Tom that Donal's attitude had helped him to get the defeat into perspective when he was motivating the team for the next game.

Donal had been reading a book called *The Art of Positive Thinking* by Geoff Thompson, and taking everything he read on board. He had moved on a long way from Harry Potter and read anything that helped him maintain an optimistic approach to his recovery.

I remember dropping him off on one occasion for a midweek session. We arrived at the pitch about half an hour before training began. It was a bleak night, the wind driving hard from the Atlantic. I looked back before I drove away and saw my son's forlorn figure, laying out cones and preparing the pitch in readiness for his squad's arrival. My eyes filled with tears as I watched him struggling against the wind but, then, I knew he'd struggled against far greater obstacles and won.

He was still growing and had to return to Cappagh Hospital to have his prosthesis extended. This was to be a relatively minor surgical procedure – compared to his previous procedures, that is – and there would be a short period of recuperation. Everything was ready, his leg iodised and so on, when Mr Dudeney asked for one more X-ray. When this was handed to him, he noticed that a screw in the original prosthesis had become detached and caused some damage. A new prosthesis was now required. While this operation was not as major as the previous one, it would be bigger than the simple adjustment we'd expected.

When Mr Dudeney came into the ward to tell him and Elma that the operation couldn't go ahead because Donal had a screw loose, Elma replied, 'Well, he gets that from his *father's* side of the family!' Mr Dudeney laughed, relieved that he was dealing with someone who, instead of castigating him, was always able to draw on her strong sense of humour at the bleakest of times.

'You are the person who operated on my son and probably saved his life,' Elma told him. 'You put so much effort into the operation that he only has a pencil-line scar on his leg. How can you expect me to be angry because Donal over-exercised his leg and carried on as if he'd never had a prosthesis inserted? This isn't your fault. It's no one's fault. It just happened.'

Elma had learned to cope with setbacks. She was strong and determined, fiercely protective of Donal yet able to stand back and allow him to make his own decisions. That was the hardest part for both of us. Letting him be. Trying not to think too far into the future. Taking one day at a time. A loose screw could be fixed. It could be joked about. The real threat was a shadow that we tried to avoid thinking about, and, instead, we celebrated each small victory achieved by Donal.

A couple of weeks later the new prosthesis arrived. The operation was successful and Donal re-started his physiotherapy to get back on his feet once again.

I look back on those years as a special time, despite the ups and downs. We finally allowed ourselves to relax, as Donal blossomed. He moved on with his coaching and began training the Under-14 squad. He was virtually their head coach and was there, no matter the weather, week in and week out.

When we enrolled him for an Irish course in the Dingle Gaeltacht, he made the friends who were going with him swear that they would not tell anyone they met there about his cancer. He stayed in a Gaeltacht house and, as is the tradition, he was looked after by the Bean an Tí. Dingle is a little over thirty minutes' drive from Blennerville, and Elma was able to keep an eye on him while he was there. Every time she arrived, he was waiting with a group of new friends, mainly female, who wanted to be driven into the town to buy their treats and toiletries. She could see he was coping without us, and the following year we enrolled him in Coláiste Íde, the college overlooking Dingle Harbour. He was delighted when he discovered that he was one of thirty boys and a hundred girls. A lot of the outdoor activities involved contact sports, like basketball, athletics, volleyball or football and were too high-risk for him. But he loved his time in the Gaeltacht, especially the céilí dancing and Irish music that's also such an important feature of the course. As well as improving his fluency in Irish, he made more new friends from different parts of Ireland. Between his time in hospitals and in the Gaeltacht, he now had a network of friends across the country and was active on Facebook and Twitter, keeping up contact with everyone.

When we heard on local radio that the committee of the London Paralympics 2012 had decided to include rowing as a sport for the first time, we felt that this was exactly what Donal needed. It was non-contact and would suit his driven personality – and the ship canal flowed by our house. He also took up kayaking and cycling, but although he enjoyed these activities, he had no interest in taking them up competitively. He knew his own mind. We could not dictate.

Chapter Twenty-Five

Career-wise, my own luck turned when I applied for a position that became available in the hotel sector, and was appointed hotel manager in the Travel Inn, Killarney. All was going well and the autumn passed without incident. After a successful six months as manager of the Travel Inn, I was asked if I would consider working an operations manager in the Maritime Hotel in Bantry. I'd be away from home for three to four nights a week, but I agreed to take on the position and see how it worked out.

Christmas 2011 was celebrated with the usual festivities and traditions. Our only worry was when Donal came down with a severe flu. He recovered, but it left him with a cough that, while not nasty enough to keep him from school, refused to clear up.

February came, and it was time to return to Dublin with Donal for his usual check-up in Crumlin. On the morning of his appointment, Elma asked me to mention his cough to Michael

Capra. 'Just in case it's significant,' she said, but I don't think either of us believed it was. Perhaps we were in denial. Our son looked the picture of good health and was full of energy. Everything was normal – except for this persistent, hacking cough.

The check-up was going well until I mentioned the cough. Instead of dismissing it, as I'd hoped he would, Michael Capra began to question Donal about the colour of the phlegm he coughed up. Were there any dark bits in it?

'Sometimes,' Donal admitted. We both felt the atmosphere in the room change. Michael immediately sought an X-ray and a chest scan. The speed with which everything started to move filled me with a horrifying sense of déjà vu. I was afraid to look at Donal. Why the rush? I knew the same question was going through his mind, but we remained outwardly calm as we walked to the radiology department.

As he waited to be called in to the X-ray area, Donal looked hard at me and asked why a cough should create such alarm. Why the fuss? I assured him it was just a precaution, but the memory of the chest X-ray that had seemed so important over two years ago kept nagging at the back of my mind. I kept it there. No way was I going to make that jump. Fate could not be so unkind, so cruel and ruthless. But I felt like throwing up when Donal went through the doors to face another scanning machine.

He emerged, pale and shaky, the scan completed. His

appetite was gone when we sat down in the hospital canteen and tried to eat some lunch. We had to see Michael in forty-five minutes. Time seemed to pass with agonising slowness. I could only imagine the thoughts churning through my son's mind as we walked back into Michael's office. Would everything be okay – or were we once again staring into the abyss?

Chapter Twenty-Six
Donal's Story

I had to go for check-ups every four months and on 15 February 2012, I went up for one with my dad. We went for a chest X-ray and took it up to my doctor. That was normal. Until he demanded that the isotope unit open, so I could have a CT scan of my chest. I took no notice. I guess I shut it out. We waited for him in a room with yellow paint on the walls. There was a bin next to me and tissues on the table. He came in and told us I had a tumour in my lung. It was back. My heart sank. My world fell apart again. I was angry. This was too much. I stood up and kicked the bin. I wanted to run. I fell to my knees in tears. I couldn't handle it. He said I would be going for surgery the week after, on 24 February. I wasn't happy to be doing this all again. They weren't able to tell if I would need chemo until after the surgery, I wasn't happy with that.

The ward hadn't changed at all. The walls were the same, the curtains were the same, the airtight windows were the same and, of course, the same empty promises given to countless dying children by countless gentlemen in suits. It really does make me ashamed of my government when they can get wages in the hundreds of thousands annually, but one of the most important children's wards in Ireland, for some of the sickest kids in Ireland, has to rely on charitable donations to buy a bucket of paint and a brush. That is one of the sickest things I have ever come across in my short lifetime here.

Chapter Twenty-Seven

Almost three-and-a-half years previously, when we'd first heard the diagnosis of osteosarcoma – and the three possible operating procedures being considered for Donal – I'd broken down in tears. Michael Capra had allowed me to cry until I recovered some composure. Then he'd stressed in no uncertain terms how important it was for me and Elma to adopt a positive attitude. The last thing Donal needed was to see his parents crack under the pressure of his treatment. He needed to believe that we were confident and optimistic that at the end of his ordeal, he would make a full recovery.

And that was what we did, no matter how grim the circumstances. Donal had struggled through his leg operation and the appalling effects of his chemo. For a brief, golden time, it seemed as if our positivity had paid off. We'd seen him adapt to his changed circumstances, grow tall and rebuild his strength, take on the challenge of rugby coaching, return to school and resume his studies, build strong and lasting friendships. He'd done everything by the book and yet – and yet ... I found it impossible to take in the enormity of what we were now hearing.

I watched the fear and anger gather on Donal's face. Unable to control his frustration, he kicked out angrily at a rubbish bin but then broke down in tears. I struggled to remain composed, although I wanted to cry with him, lash out too at the nearest object to hand. I wondered how I would break the news to Elma and Jema, to my mother and siblings, to all the people who had supported us along this torturous road. There were no words to soften the blow, nothing that would rewind the clock to those moments before this new diagnosis had been presented to us.

This time we were no longer bewildered, trying to make our way through unfamiliar hospital corridors. We were experienced veterans – but that made absolutely no difference to our grief. Our lives were in turmoil once again, and our diaries were about to be cleared. We forced ourselves to listen to what Michael was saying. Donal had battled this once before, he said. He could do so again.

Donal eventually calmed down and dried his tears. After the hospital visit, we'd planned an exciting afternoon in Dublin. He'd intended meeting Shane Jennings, the rugby player who'd kept in regular contact with him since that first visit by the lads from the Leinster team. Some days before, Donal had bought an engagement present for Shane and had hoped to give it to him. We left the hospital in a daze but Donal, to my surprise, decided he wanted to keep to our original plan.

I sent a text to Shane and warned him in advance that the test had not gone well. He was already waiting for us in a quiet corner of the popular Goat Lounge Bar in Goatstown when we arrived.

'The cancer is back,' Donal told him. 'It's gone into my lungs now.' How he kept his voice steady is beyond me, but he was able to relate the conversation that had taken place between himself and Michael.

'Hey, guys, my mother has had cancer more than once and has fought it each time,' Shane said. 'You're in the second row now and the fight starts right now. You have to be positive to beat this thing!' The conversation continued in this vein and I saw Donal draw strength from Shane's conviction. It was like a pep talk before a tough, hard match and Donal responded, his natural optimism overcoming his dread. Yet none of us was in any doubt about the struggle that lay ahead.

Elma believes it was Donal's courageous attitude that brought us through his cancer. I agree with her. If he had not been so positive, we simply would not have been able to mount our defences against this second onslaught.

I was taking care of Donal and I asked Dr Capra to phone Elma with the sad news. She was at work and totally unprepared for such devastating information. She was waiting when we returned home. As soon as Donal saw her, he broke down again. She too was weeping as she reached for him and held him tightly to her. Sometimes, that's all you can do. And, sometimes, that's all that's needed.

Once the shock of this devastating news had been absorbed, Donal lost no time contacting Paul O'Connell. Paul, speaking privately to me, asked why Donal's operation would not take place for another week. Was it a question of finance? If so, that problem could be sorted out immediately. I reassured Paul that we were okay. Donal was in no immediate danger. If he was to receive such instant attention, it would mean the cancellation of another child's operation.

Donal's operation took place as arranged. Whenever I closed my eyes, I visualised this vicious alien clawing at my son's lung, spitting and secreting its spores, as it tried to remain attached to his body. After it was over, we saw a ravaged child with tubes everywhere. He was assisted in his breathing by pumps and was so seriously ill that Elma, when she phoned me one evening, admitted that if he was to suffer any more, she would ask God to take him and give him peace. I knew she was close to breaking point by that stage. To be willing to endure the loss of her beloved son, so that his suffering could be alleviated, was the greatest sacrifice she could make.

Slowly, painfully, Donal came back to us. The care and attention he received from the staff in Crumlin would not have been bettered anywhere. Gradually, as he recovered, visitors were allowed to see him. Donal's dislike of hospital food was legendary by this stage and when Donal, his namesake uncle, and his cousins Amy, James and Christine came to visit, they brought homemade salads, sandwiches and delicious desserts. His cousins, all around his own age, would sit on his bed as they all tucked into the food and talked non-stop about films, sport, clothes and music. Donal's taste in music was eclectic and individualistic. His choices ranged from Coldplay to The Dubliners, Makem and Clancy to The Coronas – he also followed other obscure bands who took his fancy. He enjoyed the English pop band McFly and was a fan of the American rapper Macklemore, when he had very few Irish followers. Donal had in fact bought a ticket for Macklemore's sell-out gig in the O2, but sadly had passed away before he could go. Kieran, my brother, and his two sons Sean and Ronan, were also regular visitors and these young cousins were a welcome substitute for Donal's Kerry friends who lived so far away. They made his days seem shorter and he was always delighted to see them.

He kept in touch with his heroes and their positive influence helped him when things were really grim. If Paul O'Connell (or 'Paulie' as he called him) and Shane texted that they were going to drop in to see him, Donal made sure he had a shower and his teeth were brushed before their arrival, even though he might have spent the morning vomiting his guts up. They had an influence on him way beyond what we, as mere parents, could achieve.

On one occasion when he was still linked up to tubes, he had two visitors: his close friend from Kerry, John Kelly, and Paul, who was in Dublin to play in the Six Nations against Italy. We were relaxed and chatting about the upcoming Six Nations, when three doctors arrived to remove the final tube that was attached to Donal. We asked if we should leave, but he wanted us to remain with him.

The doctors proceeded to remove the tube, which was about 40 centimetres inside Donal's body. Paul, looking stoic, was standing on my right-hand side. John, who was on my left, decided to film the procedure on his mobile phone. Inch by inch, the tube was eased out from Donal's lung. He was trying to be as brave as possible but it was obviously extremely painful, and the two lads on either side of me were growing paler by the minute. I looked from one to the other and quickly moved to the other side of John. If he fainted, I could catch him but if the big fellow went down, I'd be in trouble if I tried to stop his fall. How could I explain to Declan Kidney that his captain had fainted in the Children's Hospital in Crumlin before a vital Six Nations match? Thankfully, I didn't have to make that call, but it was a very shaken captain of the Irish rugby team who left Donal's bedside that day.

Chapter Twenty-Eight
Donal's Story

I broke down the morning of my operation. I didn't want to do it because it meant I would be going back to that life, the life I swore I left behind, the life I was promised I wouldn't see again. They tried to sedate me but I refused because taking that medicine would be like accepting it was real and I couldn't do that. Eventually I was sedated and that was it. The next thing I remember was waking up in intensive care with my mom next to me. She was crying.

'Did everything go okay?' I asked.

She wiped her eyes. 'Yeah, everything's okay,' she said unconvincingly.

'Why are you—?' Then it hit me. 'I need chemo, don't I?'

She began to cry again. 'Yes,' she said.

I didn't know what to do. My mom never cries in front of me. I knew there was more. I wanted to hold her but I couldn't move. I have to show her I'm okay.

'I'm okay, Mom. I'll be fine. Don't cry. I can do it again,' I lied.

The next day I realised I was back to where I was three years ago. In intensive care, with an epidural, two drainage tubes in my lung, countless cannulas, a catheter and a pain tube in my throat.

I was going to march through this. I was getting out of here and going home before the chemo. That's all I wanted. I met with my surgeon that day. It turned out the tumour was three times the size they thought it was. It was twelve centimetres. They had to remove half my lung with it.

I got started on the rehab. This time she said we were going to walk two doors down the corridor, a space of ten metres. It wasn't long enough: half the corridor – 30 metres – would do me. I was leaving Friday and to do that, the doctors had to see I was okay. I left Friday.

I had ten days at home and I had to decide if I was going to do the chemo or not. If I did, I was told it would be very tough and they don't know how long it will go on for. If I didn't, [the cancer] would come back and I might not survive. For those ten days, I didn't know if I wanted to be Donal. I wanted to be something more. I wanted to leave Donal behind with a bang. I was told to do some crazy things, but in the end I chose to be Donal because when I made up my mind, either way, I was going to have to leave him behind and I wanted to appreciate everything he had as a normal teenager. I've met some people who have no idea how lucky their lives are. And I wasn't going to finish without appreciating what I had.

I spent those ten days with my friends and family. On the Saturday before my chemo, I went to Cork with my best friend and his brother. I nearly had another breakdown on the train. They saved me. Straight away I was on the phone to another good friend in Limerick and he helped me make up my mind about the chemo, and I owe it all to those three guys. They're all like brothers to me now.

Chapter Twenty-Nine

Once again, we faced into the horrors of chemotherapy. This time the treatments were five days on and two weeks off. I would take Donal to Dublin on a Sunday evening or early Monday morning, and the treatment would start immediately his blood results came in. He would have the chemo until Thursday evening with a twenty-four-hour wash-out, and return home on Friday. I would be in St John's with him until Wednesday and then head to work in Bantry after a brief lunch with Elma, as we passed over duties. Once again, we had to cope with fleeting meetings, intense conversations over the phone and an overriding sense of anxiety dominating our days.

Donal had grown in height since his previous time in hospital and was now six feet three inches tall. Because of his size and weight, he was put on an adult dose of etoposide. This drug had worked well in his previous treatment, but the new dosage made him very sleepy. He refused to be doped out of his head. An alternative was tried, but the effects were the same. The third treatment seemed to work, at least initially. But on the third night, all hell broke loose.

A new patient had just been admitted St John's Ward and was sharing a room with Donal. I'd tried to show his mother, who was a nurse, how we could best manage to live together as strangers in such close proximity. I was sleeping overnight in the ward with Donal, and she would be doing the same with her son. We fell into a fitful sleep but Donal awoke at midnight. He needed to use the urine bottle but was unable to control his spasmodic jerking as he tried to pee. I did my best to help him, but he developed a convulsion worse than any epileptic seizure I'd ever witnessed.

Emergency buttons were pressed, nurses came, but were helpless because of Donal's size and spasms. A kick or a blow from him would have sent them to the ground. All I could do was stand behind him and protect him from banging off any of the instruments or objects surrounding his bed. I screamed and prayed for a doctor to come and administer something, anything, to stop this seizure. Our new neighbours were given the worst possible introduction to the ward that night. There was nothing to shield that mother or her child from this demonstration of the side effects that sometimes followed a bout of chemotherapy. Later, when the nurse manager took me aside to discuss what happened, I broke down in tears. I was physically exhausted and emotionally devastated. I had really thought we were going to lose him that time and I was not ready for that – not ready at all.

I told the nurse that I'd always been extremely sensitive to sedative drugs. Donal was still practically a child, despite his size. I suggested that, as he had done so well on etoposide two years previously, they should try putting him back on a child's dose. This was done and he remained under observation for the rest of the week. Thankfully, there was no repeat of that frightening seizure.

Before we left at the end of the week, one of the team said that mothers usually had an instinctive knowledge about what their sick children needed. Sometimes this could be at variance with medical opinion – it would be an arrogant doctor who did not listen to a mother's concerns. Fathers could also get it right on occasions, she added – and that's what I'd done in this case. It was a small sliver of comfort to take with me, as Donal and I headed once again for the road home.

While he was undergoing his chemotherapy, John Kelly, who had recorded the memorable tube-pulling episode, now worked with Donal on a video called *My Struggle with Cancer*, which they uploaded on to YouTube. Once again, Donal had lost his hair but this time, unlike the previous occasion when he was convinced everyone would be staring at him, he had no problem going public. This video was filled with hope but did not shy away from the side effects of Donal's treatment. It is one of the most moving YouTube clips I've ever watched. In fact, the Children's Medical & Research Foundation for Crumlin Hospital now use it on a Donal Walsh fundraising website, along with a number of interviews he did for them during his time in hospital.

In June Donal left St John's as a patient and headed home to do his Junior Certificate examination. Because his blood counts were still low, a special examination centre was set up at home for him. The invigilator came by each day and Donal sat every exam under the same strict conditions as those that operated in the classroom. His blood cell count went down during the second English paper, which meant he had to finish early and go to Kerry General for a transfusion. As a result, he missed out on his German and Geography exams the following day – but, considering the trauma of the previous four months, it was an achievement in itself that he was able to sit any of the papers.

Chapter Thirty
Donal's Story

Four months in there, is what I was told at the start, so four months is what I was aiming for. The first treatment was a week long, inside in the ward. It was also Cheltenham race week. All the information we had gotten four years ago was being thrown back at us – it was like nothing had changed but a few inches in height. My Hickman was put back in the same place, I was put into the same beds next to the same machines and next to very similar families.

The week seemed to be a short one, even though it was very tough. I was using Cheltenham as an excuse to get up every morning and it gave me a distraction while my body was being persecuted by the two chemos again. My mom and I left Crumlin at the end of that week on St Patrick's Day and we were getting home, no matter what parade got in our way!

It hurt every time I had to leave home and such a beautiful part of the world, to be locked up in that cage, but it had to be done. While I was there, my mom noticed that I was getting a lot of headaches and I was losing memory, so immediately they had me do a brain scan, which came back clear. That meant that it must have been one of the chemos. So they stopped the ifosfamide for what was left in that week and I was home a day early as a result of it.

I had three weeks at home to recover before my next bout of chemo. I was back to the old routine, with my injection every morning and the vomiting bowl following me round the house. But now I had to put on a show because my friends couldn't see the sick Donal. They obviously knew, along with half the town, that my cancer was back and they knew that I was going to be sick after my treatments. But they're still only teenagers. I would make sure that I was able for their visits and that I could do most of the things they did, but sometimes I'd have to use an excuse – like I was out of breath because of my lung or my knee was sore. But we had some good laughs about the cancer as well, they'd always have a joke or two to crack and I even let them shave my hair off one night, which was a funny experience. It's hard to call them 'friends'. When they spend every day with you, they become family.

It was my third week for chemo. They told me they had changed the medications like the anti-sickness so I shouldn't feel any more of the headaches, yet after two days of chemo I still struggled to remember who my mom was. Something clicked with my mom that she had seen this before in her mother, my gran, where she had steroid psychosis. This meant as a result of too much steroids we couldn't remember family and who we were. The doctors adjusted this medicine and all my memory came back.

During my two-week breaks, I would have spent most of the time recovering while my friends were at school. I had one friend who came around every day after school and made me smile.

That was John. He visited me in hospital and made me laugh, even though it hurt like hell. We ended up like brothers throughout it all. Then there's Cormac, Hugh and James, my three best friends from school – they supported me through everything and visited me as much as they could while studying for their exams. I was also trying to study for my Junior Cert as best as I could, but I could only make it into school for one week while I was at home. This made it difficult at times but I had huge support from my school and they helped me to do as much work as I could at home.

It soon began to dawn on me I was coming up to my last chemo session before they decided if I was finished with it or not: the plan was for me to finish the fourth chemo and go home to recover before they would do a scan which would give me all the results. I went for my last chemo and finished my last ifosfamide and etoposide before the scan. The chemos hadn't worn me out as physically this time as they did the first time: I had only lost a stone-and-a-half in weight and my appetite wasn't as badly affected. While I was recovering, I began to feel awful negative. With the scan approaching, all I could think about was how the chemos didn't affect my body as badly as they should have, like the first time. The more I thought about it, the more I realised I didn't get sick enough to kill off all the good cells and the bad cells, but the doctors reassured me that because they were two different chemotherapy combinations, there would be two different results and I had to remain positive for the scan the following week.

The scan was booked for Friday, 15 June 2012 – my sixteenth birthday. I drove up to Dublin with my mom and sister. After the scan, we came home for the weekend and waited for the results.

On the Monday, the Junior Cert exams, which I sat at home, had finished so I went to James's house with Cormac and Hugh, where we were going to watch Ireland in Euro 2012.

My phone rang: it was my mom. She said, 'The results are back from the scan and it was all-clear, you don't need any more chemo.' I couldn't believe it – that all I had thought over the last few weeks and all I had gone through over the past few months was over! I spent the summer travelling between Bantry and Tralee. I spent the time in Bantry with my cycling coach, James Cleary and the rest of the time in Tralee, working my ass off in the gym and on the bike. I even changed my diet to help me build my strength and fitness levels.

I returned to school in September and had gotten into a daily routine of an early start at 7 a.m. to get my food ready for the day, go to school, go straight to the gym or go for a cycle (I had reached up to 60 kilometres at the time), come and study and then some weeknights, coach youth rugby. My life seemed to be perfect. I had everything I ever wanted and it couldn't have gone any better.

Chapter Thirty-One

Where did he get his strength? His determination? Donal was no saint, that's for sure. He was as mischievous as any other teenager, capable of strong opinions, occasional brooding silences, bursting with determination and an energy that he used to the full – and, alongside all of that, he had a deep spirituality. He was not self-conscious about it, nor did he preach his own beliefs to those around him. This was his private conversation with God and his faith sat easily on his shoulders.

Donal had been baptised a Catholic and his faith had been nurtured by us, his family, and his close-knit community. But his spirituality went beyond ritual and prayer, although he believed in both. During the years of his illness, he built up a number of spiritual relationships with our local priests and a man called John Delaney. John is recognised throughout Ireland as a man of prayer. A very busy person, he still found time to be with Donal throughout his illness. John explained to him that his own gift of healing came directly from a power greater than himself. If Donal was to be healed, then that healing would be part of God's plan and John was there to help Donal accept whatever route his journey took. They became good friends, relaxed in each other's company, whether they were having a conversation or praying. Donal was still a typical teenager. He liked his mobile and his Wii, his games and matches, his drums and hanging out with his friends in the den. Yet he had no difficulty merging his spirituality with the more worldly side of his personality.

He attended school when he was strong enough. One day during English class, Des Healy, his English teacher, asked the class to write an essay on something big that had occurred in their lives. Donal began to write a short essay about his battle with cancer. Once he started, the words flowed from him. All his pent-up fears, his determination and courage poured onto the page. Des was deeply moved when he read it and asked Donal's permission to show the essay to the rest of the class. He then phoned us to see if that was okay. He wanted the students to take it home and read it then put it away, to be read again at some future time when they were having a really bad day.

'It's an astonishing piece of writing from such a young boy,' Des said, and I agreed with him when I read it. Seeing Donal's thoughts laid out so bluntly brought home the enormity of his own anguish and the suffering being experienced by other young patients who were undergoing the same ordeal.

The essay was subsequently published in the CBS Year Book, where I hope it will be read by the students of the future, and inspire in them that same determination to live life to its fullest degree, whatever the odds.

Weather-wise, the summer was disappointing. The sun was an infrequent visitor, but Donal was anxious to get back to full fitness as soon as possible. He also resumed his earlier fundraising activities. He'd seen too much, heard too many stories and, having returned there so recently and found things exactly the same, he renewed his efforts to help with the planned redevelopment of St John's Ward.

The support he got from the people of Tralee and surrounding areas was amazing. They ran marathons, climbed mountains, baked cakes, organised quizzes and bungee jumps, ran 'Bald' or 'Blue' days, and undertook a host of other activities that raised €50,000 over a six-month period.

The Maritime Hotel in Bantry, where I now work, has excellent gym and spa facilities, as well as a swimming pool. When Donal stayed with me in the hotel for a weekend, I introduced him to James, our Leisure Club Manager. James worked out a training programme for him and set Donal a series of goals to help improve his breathing and increase his stamina. One such goal was to get back on his bike and start cycling. This would be beneficial for his endurance breathing, James said, and the idea immediately appealed to Donal.

Impatient as ever, he now wanted a new racing bike. Secretly, he set himself the goal of participating in the Ring of Kerry Charity Cycle the following year. Yes, our competitive son was back in action. He rushed out to choose his racing bike and settled on a bright yellow, stainless steel model that was a bit on the heavy side, I thought. James also hoped he would opt for a lighter, hybrid version but Donal knew exactly what he wanted. Within weeks of starting his training programme, he was doing 60-kilometre cycles, three or four times a week. He was also back in the gym, pumping light weights and eating like an athlete.

The problems we'd had persuading him to eat during his previous bout of cancer no longer existed. He ate everything that was placed in front of him, in an effort to keep up his weight. He talked about doing the Tour de France at some point, not as a para-athlete but as a normal racer. While I smiled, I also knew he was serious. If all it took was determination or ambition to get to that level of fitness, then he would be doing the Tour at some point in the future.

I'd heard about the CROSS Rugby Legends Cycle in aid of cancer research. The cycle is done in stages from Mizen Head to Malin Head, and I introduced Donal to the idea of doing one of the stages. He jumped at the chance of joining the Legends. He trained hard with James so that he could do the Kerry stage from Moll's Gap to Killarney, then lead the group into Tralee. And that is exactly what he did. With his prosthetic knee and two-thirds lung capacity, he cycled into Tralee to a rapturous welcome home.

Looking back now, I realise he wanted to cram every experience he could into his life. The second bout of cancer had shaken him badly, and he must have known that his future hung in the balance. He now decided to learn to drive. As I was working in Bantry and away from home for part of the week, it was his uncle Brian who took over and taught him. Brian was a patient teacher and Donal was soon driving around the family farm. Jema laughs when she remembers how he begged her not to do her driving test until he had passed his.

We planned to take a holiday in late October 2012. This would probably be our last chance to holiday together as a family, now that Jema was starting college. She had successfully completed her Leaving Certificate with the necessary points for the course she wanted to do, which was a TV, Radio and New Media Studies degree in IT Tralee. Donal had also been successful in his Junior Cert with two Bs, three Cs, three Ds and an F – not a bad result from someone who had missed out on half of his second English Paper, nearly three months of classes, and was undergoing chemotherapy at the time he sat the examination. We were proud of both of our children, and the holiday would give us an opportunity to relax before the next round of check-ups for Donal, which were due to take place in November.

He took out his bike one evening in September for his regular ride from Tralee to Killorglin and back again, a distance of about 50 kilometres. He was wearing his high visibility jacket and had lights on his bike and his arms. He also had the right of way, but a car came from a side turning and collided with him. He was knocked from his bike and collapsed on the road. The horrified driver rang the guards and Elma received a call on Donal's mobile from the garda who attended the scene. She was terrified as she drove to see Donal in the Accident and Emergency ward in Kerry General.

Although shaken by the fall, Donal seemed fine. He'd suffered a slightly dislocated shoulder, some cracked ribs and lots of bruises. His only consolation was that, for once, he was in Kerry

General for something other than his cancer. Apart from these minor injuries, and his shock, he seemed okay. X-rays were taken and once the doctors were assured he was not suffering from concussion, they reluctantly, at his insistence, discharged him that same evening. He had seen enough of the inside of hospitals and had no wish to spend an extra minute in another one, if he could possibly avoid it.

Chapter Thirty-Two
Donal's Story

One day in September, I went on a cycle route of 55 kilometres, and on the way back, coming through a small village, I was hit by a car. I was hit on the left and landed on that side as I had flipped so many times in the air. I couldn't move and by the time someone had gotten to me, they stopped me from moving, in case I made any injuries worse. The ambulance and gardai arrived and I was brought to Kerry General Hospital. All I was thinking was the worst, but thankfully it never came to that. A few broken ribs and bad internal bruising on my shoulder and leg, but I walked out of there the following evening.

This crash had me thinking – I didn't realise how much I loved training. It was what made me happy in my life because it made me feel alive. Those pains and aches from training in the gym and all those cuts and bruises from the bike, they were all signs that I was alive and healthy and I loved it, because it showed people how far I'd come. From being four-and-a-half stone and learning how to walk again, to having half my lung removed and having the scare of losing my memory – to being able to go to the gym

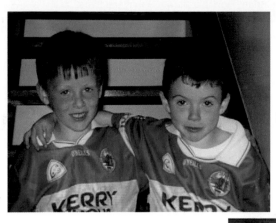

Donal and his best friend Cian (aged 7)

Donal (aged 4) and Jema (aged 6)

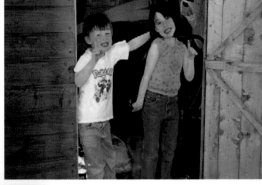

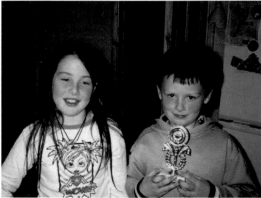

Jema (aged 10) and Donal (aged 8) with first 'Naries' trophy

Jema (aged 5), Elma and Donal (aged 3) on family picnic at Glentenassig Woods

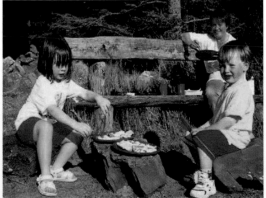

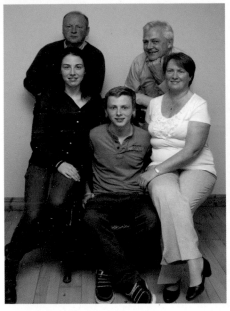

Brian, Fionnbar, Jema, Donal and Elma,
November 2012
(Photographs by Mary O'Connell)

Donal and Mom, November 2012

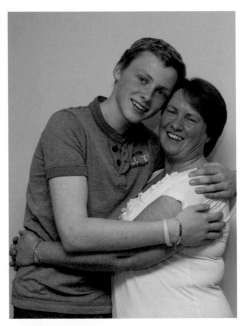

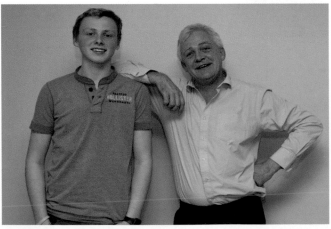

Donal and Fionnbar,
November 2012

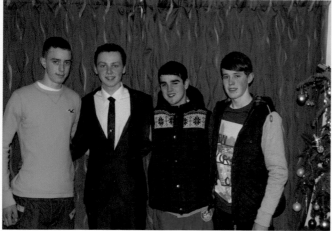

William, Donal, Cormac and Ger, Debs Night, January 2013

Donal, Hugh, Cormac and James in Ballyheigue for helicopter ride

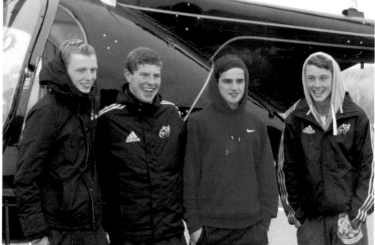

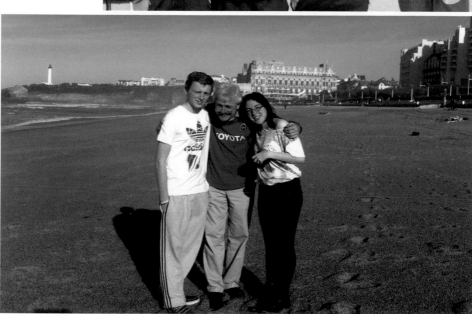

Donal, Fionnbar and Jema in Biarritz on the way home from Lourdes

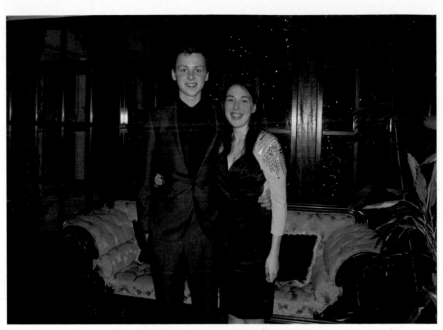

Donal and Jema, NYE 2012, Ballygarry House

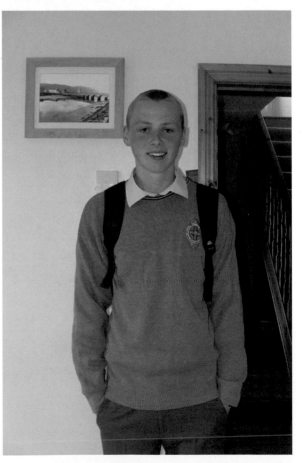

Donal returning to 5th Year
at school, September 2012

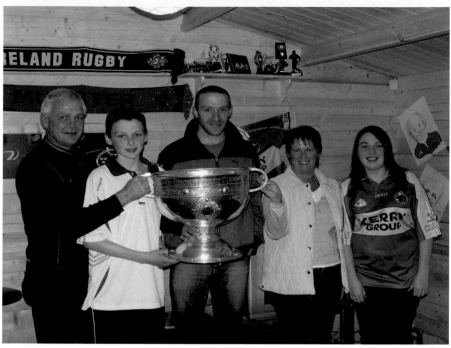

Fionnbar, Donal, Tommy Griffin, Elma, Jema and Sam in The Shed

Donal's rugby squad, West Munster League winners 2011

Back row: Fionnbar, Gary Ellis, Josh Barnes, Sean Browne, Gerard Brown, Donal O'Connell,
Michael Mulally, Glen Brazil, James D. O'Connor, Darren McKenzie Vass, Ciarán Ó Nualláin
Front row: Mick Flanagan, James O'Connor, Cillian White, Jake Foley, Liam Gannon,
Ciarán Flanagan, John Kelly, Seán Doyle & Donal
(Photograph by David Condon)

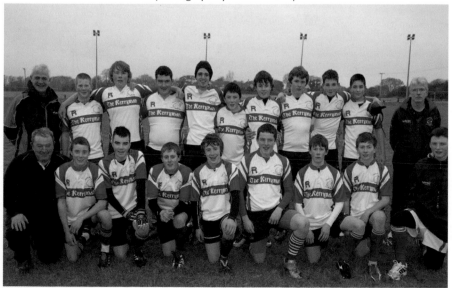

Anthony (Axel) Foley
and Donal

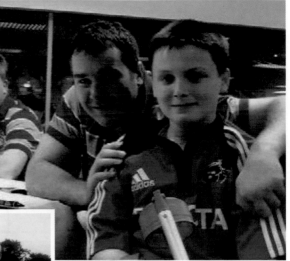

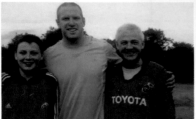

Paul O'Connell, Donal and Fionnbar

Donal with Alan Quinlan,
October 2008 in Thomond Park
v Glasgow Warriors

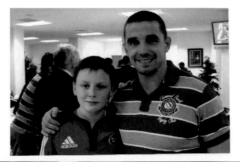

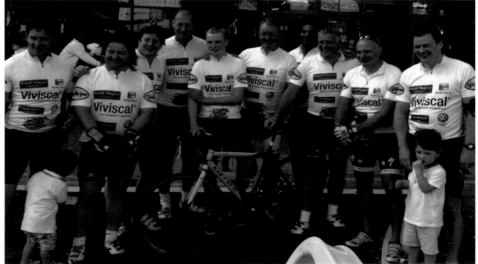

Donal with the Cross Rugby Legends, September 2012

Left to right: David Wallace, Shane Byrne, Paul Wallace, Paddy Johns, Donal, Mick Galwey,
Colin Charvis, Scott Hastings, Denis McBride, Richard Wallace

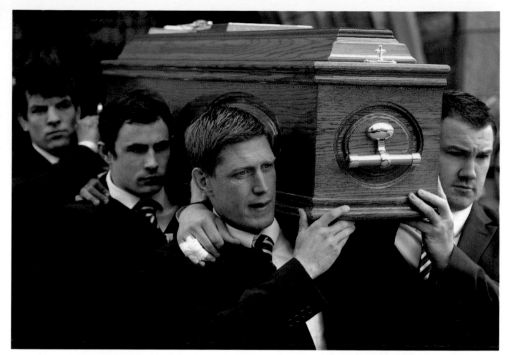

Donncha O'Callaghan, J.J. Hanrahan, Ronan O'Gara and Damien Varley
from the Munster rugby team carry Donal's coffin
(Photographs by Domnick Walsh)

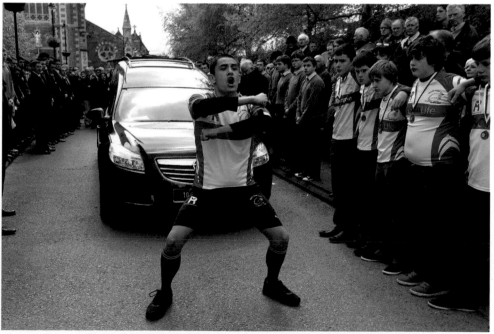

Danny Cournane performs the Haka on the day of Donal's funeral

Fionnbar and Elma at the Rehab
People of the Year Awards 2013
where Donal was honoured with
a posthumous award
(Photograph by Robbie Reynolds)

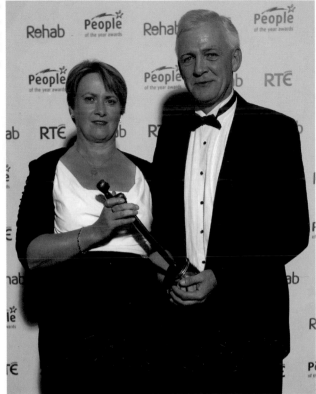

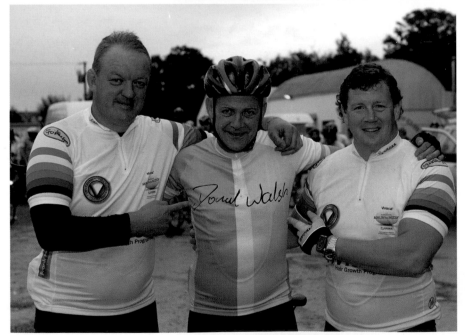

Fionnbar, with Mick Galwey and Paul Wallace at the CrossDonalsMountain Challenge,
the Kerry stage of the CROSS Cycle Challenge, 2013
(Photograph by Domnick Walsh)

every day, cycle 60 kilometres and love every second of it: this was what kept me going. And what made it even better was no one expected it. Anyone who saw me in hospital during those times couldn't believe how far I'd come. It was like a miracle.

For the few weeks after the crash, I was plagued by minor injuries and setbacks in the gym, in particular my right shoulder, which was the opposite one to which the crash affected. So about a month after the crash, my mom took me to A & E one morning. The doctor that saw me was the same doctor that treated me for the crash. They X-rayed my shoulder and put it down to a torn muscle from over-exercising.

So life went back to normal, school with Cormac, James and Hugh, and John every other spare second I had. I had the best friends anyone could ask for and I knew it, but had no way to show it, but I tried to be as best a friend as I could be for them.

The pain wasn't improving much over the weeks I was resting it. With the check-up in Crumlin approaching, my mind wasn't at ease anymore.

Chapter Thirty-Three

In mid-October 2012 we received an invitation to attend the official launch of the Crumlin Hospital renovation project. Donal, along with the other fundraisers, was invited to a celebratory lunch, to thank him for the €50,000 he had raised for the hospital. He had an appointment to see Michael Capra in November, but we had rescheduled it so that it could be done on the same day as the lunch. We were looking forward to our family holiday and it would be a relief to have Donal's check-up out of the way.

Donal and I both dressed smartly for the launch and were leaving the house when Elma mentioned Donal's shoulder. It should be checked out, she said. Just in case ... It wasn't hard to guess what was on her mind and that chilled feeling crept over me again. I convinced myself we were overreacting. We had the accident to explain the pain and Donal was looking amazingly fit and healthy.

At the check-up appointment that morning, which was before the lunch, Michael called us into his office and we went through the usual detailed questions about how everything was progressing. The chest X-rays that had been taken were clear. Things seemed to be okay. We were looking forward to enjoying lunch and getting back on the road to Tralee as quickly as possible. Then I mentioned the accident to Michael, and Donal admitted that his shoulder was still giving him so much trouble, he had been unable to get back up on his bike. Michael said there was no reason for any of his patients to be in any unnecessary pain. He would organise a scan and if something needed to be done, he would get the right people to look at the shoulder. He rang down to the Radiology department and asked if the CT scanner was available. It was due to be serviced that day, he was told, and the technician had just arrived to begin his work. Michael contacted the head of Radiology, however, and had the service stopped. I fought back my apprehension and convinced myself it was just a precaution. Michael was not going to take any chances with Donal and it was important to get everything done while we were in Dublin.

After the scan was completed, we attended the lunch. This should have been a proud moment for Donal. All his fundraising efforts had paid off. But I could see he was nervous. He knew the unexpected could come like a bolt from the blue at any time, and was experienced enough to see behind the professional masks of the medical personnel who looked after him. The speeches were over and we had just started our meal when my mobile rang. My heart plummeted when I realised it was Michael Capra. I went outside to take his call and knew before he spoke that the news was stark. How much worse could things get?

Michael was calm as he warned me in advance to compose myself. I was to return with Donal to his office as soon as lunch was over. The cancer was back and it was necessary to review everything. I called Elma immediately and tried to prepare her for what was to come. But how do you prepare anyone for the prospect of such news? You can't. All we could do was breathe slowly and hold on to our sanity, because no matter how awful we felt, we needed to be strong.

My lunch was tasteless. How I kept the food down is a mystery. Or how I conversed intelligently with those around me. Donal filled my eyes. He was all that mattered. How would he cope with the news he was about to receive? Over those four years of his illness, I'd watched him mature, grow strong again, live life to its fullest, always believing there was a future to be prized.

Chapter Thirty-Four
Donal's Story

My check-up was scheduled for 19 November, but because €50,000 was raised in my name for Crumlin and the ward, I was invited up for a charitable launch in October – so I had my check-up changed to match them both on 16 October.

So me and my dad set off. We arrived early at 9 a.m., so we could be first in and first out, hopefully. We took our chairs in the waiting room and I was weighed and had my blood pressure taken. Soon after, we were called into Dr Capra's office. My dad and him had their usual slagging match and then he started his routine exam. It seemed to all be going fine until I brought up my shoulder. I explained to him everything from the crash and he still wasn't happy. He rang down to the CT department but they were closed for repairs. He then ordered that it be opened for my shoulder scan. That's when I began to worry. I did the scan but the results wouldn't be for an hour or two, perfect for us because it fitted the time of the charity launch. We went over, and it was a weird experience because the room was full of businessmen giving speeches – but all I heard was white noise, nothing. I couldn't even concentrate on worrying, just waiting for the phone call to bring us back for the results. The call came.

I sat back in the waiting room with my dad. Dr Capra called our names from the door of the waiting room, and when I walked over, he said, 'We've been on this road too many times, eh?'

That was it. My heart sank. I didn't know whether to follow them to his office or run out the front door. 'It's bad news, isn't it?' I asked.

'I'm afraid so,' he confirmed.

I didn't break down this time, I shed a tear and asked what the prognosis was now. He said he couldn't confirm a plan of treatment yet but more than likely, it would involve some form of surgery and chemo treatments – but that it was unlikely it would work because it had failed twice before. And if it did work, it wouldn't stay away.

'So if it doesn't kill me this time, it will the next?' I asked bluntly.

'Well, the cancer has become immune to the treatments, so eventually it will, yes,' he answered.

That's when I burst into tears, that's when I realised I was hanging from a building, relying on my little finger. I couldn't get over it – I was so healthy, I had changed everything to avoid this, to avoid cancer but it still caught me. That trip home was the most heart-breaking, telling my mom and my sister while we were all in tears, and other people I loved, like John and the lads, that the cancer had caught me and it looked like it was going to kill me.

We arrived home four hours later to a house full of support, everyone had come out. That week was a blur to me. After letting the news out that the cancer was back, the amount of support that I got was crazy. I didn't need any of that chin-up bullshit, because I had all the positivity and strength and support I needed to get through this ten times over, but it still felt like a mountain I couldn't climb. Nonetheless God had given me hiking boots, so I might as well start climbing.

Chapter Thirty-Five

The boy who entered Michael's office that day walked out a man. He was facing the ultimate reality. The toughest test life had thrown at him, and his questions to Michael had been direct.

'If it's only one tumour, what can you do?'

'What are my chances if there is more than one?'

And that last, terrifying, unavoidable question: 'Realistically, how long do I have?'

How different they were, these stark questions, to the innocent ones he had asked in Cappagh Hospital when he was twelve years old and scared that he might not awaken from an anaesthetic.

How long do I have? That question trembled in the air. I didn't want to hear the answer but I knew I must endure it. And, somehow, we did find endurance when Michael informed us that Donal had between three to six months before his cancer finally won out. It had struck in a completely new area and there was little hope that it would not be found elsewhere. From now on, we had to depend on faith and whatever hope we could draw from our prayers, and the prayers of those around us. We were no longer staring into the abyss. We had fallen headlong into it. Donal's medical team had already used the Rolls Royce of chemotherapies. The other available ones were of lesser quality and would not have any effect. He would not be put through any unnecessary suffering with no gain at the end. From now on, it was pain management. They would keep their international contacts on the alert, to see if there was anything else that might offer hope. But we needed to be realistic. I saw the grief on Michael's face when he answered Donal's questions. To fight so hard to save a life and have to break the news that it has come to naught must be a searing task.

An early Christmas might be a good idea, Michael advised us, before we left. An early Christmas! We were in the middle of October. Christmas was only about nine weeks away as it was.

The road from Dublin to Kerry was all too familiar to us: home to hospital, hospital to home. Elma and I had driven it in states of extreme distress, in a fever of hope, in despair and optimism. We had run the gauntlet of emotions but we were never certain of the future. Now, all that had changed. The future was decided. This road I wished had been less travelled opened before Donal and me, in a blur of traffic. I don't know how I drove on that fateful day. Madness. But I had to bring my son home to his mother's arms.

'You'll still fight this,' I told Donal as the miles flashed by. And I really believed we could, despite all the evidence to the contrary. One heard such stories. A magic bullet. The miracle cure. Donal was a fighter. My thoughts veered from hopelessness to a crazed belief in the impossible.

'It's not over yet,' he agreed.

'Not by a long shot,' I reassured him.

And that was how we comforted each other, with clichés and platitudes because, sometimes, when the shock is extreme, it takes time to delve bravely down into the truth.

Elma was waiting with Jema, the house full of family and supporters, their tears dried as they prepared to greet Donal. How do you deal with such an obscenity? And what was happening was obscene. I wanted to rail to the heavens against it, but the finality of Michael's verdict had left me bereft of fight.

Over the following days we made no attempt to check our tears. They flowed every time Elma and I tried to discuss what was happening. Our hearts and our spirits were broken. It was Donal who lifted us out of the abyss. He was not going anywhere without a fight. No deadlines, he said, as our extended family, neighbours and friends circled the wagons, as they had done when he was twelve and just starting off on this journey.

'What do you need?' they asked. 'We want to help. Tell us how!'

The kindness of people and their resourcefulness was something we found remarkable at this time, but we were too dazed to know what we needed. Catriona, our social worker, sat us down and made us focus on this new reality. She advised us to take whatever support was being offered. Donal's time was short and we needed to create everlasting memories for ourselves, his friends and extended family. Most importantly, we had to make his remaining time with us as entertaining and engrossing as possible. He had always been the first up with fundraising ideas – now we had to let others raise funds for him.

The support we received went far beyond our expectations. In work, the personnel department became involved soon after the news broke. They called me into the office one day and told me that everyone in the company wanted to help. I was still in a relatively new position, with over five hundred co-workers, and I was deeply touched by their concern. I was unsure what they could do but told them about the financial plans people were already making for Donal. They came back a few days later with an idea. They would offer the staff the option of surrendering the minimum of a half-day of their holidays in support of Donal. In the end they committed around 1,500 hours from the group. If you take that at minimum wages, you can guess the size of the figure that was offered to us. This company was large but it was strong on family values and this was an example of its humanity. Casey & Co., where Elma worked, and where her job had been kept open each time she had to leave to look after Donal, were also extremely generous in their support. Tralee RFC and Kerins O'Rahillys GAA club organised fundraising events and, as always, our extended family showed that same generosity of spirit.

With advice from friends, we put a plan into place to create the memories we would cherish when Donal was no longer with us. Some of the funds would be used for Donal's care when that harrowing time came. Whatever money was left after he died would be used to allow us, as a family, to take a short break. We would need to gather our energy for the struggle ahead, as we adjusted to life without him. The rest would go to the Kare4Kids and the Palliative Care Unit in Kerry General Hospital. But that was in the bleak future and, for now, our focus was on filling Donal's life with fun and excitement. Party time had started and was to continue for as long as possible. We couldn't bear to think there would be an end. No matter how hard we tried to accept the inevitable, it simply didn't make sense to anyone but Donal. He refused to be defeated and we – his parents and sister – seeing his determination, wondered if a miracle was possible: if sheer fortitude and mind power could triumph over death.

Chapter Thirty-Six
Donal's Story

We were called up for scans the following Thursday. Two of my friends, John and Cassie, came with me. They were a distraction for most of the day until I had to meet my doctor, and he bluntly gave us the grim news again. On the way home, I stopped in Portlaoise to meet with prayer minister John Delaney. He has been a very strong part of my faith and on that night we prayed together. I thought to myself that if this was what God wants me to do – if he wants me to fight cancer, if he wants me to be a symbol to other people, or if he just wants me to die – then I guess I'll strap up my hiking boots and get to the top of this mountain.

Two days later, my dad, John and I were sent to Dublin for a PET scan. There was a four-day wait before any results came back. I was upstairs when the call came. I walked in on my mom on the phone. My uncle Brian tried to distract me by bringing me out of the room, but I knew straight away what it was, and I wasn't leaving the room until the phone call was over. My mom hung up in tears and started to explain that there were six tumours, all growing aggressively and no treatment options available.

I didn't know what to do. I went down to my friend Vicky's house and Cassie was there too, while my mom told my sister. They were heartbroken, but it still hadn't hit me. I went back home and rang John Kelly. We spent a good while on the phone but it didn't seem real to us. James, Hugh and Cormac found it so hard to believe because I was so fit at the time.

So we thought about what to do next. It wasn't the logical thing but all we could think of was a party with all my best friends and then to hit the town afterwards.

After that week, it was mid-term and everyone had a few days to let it sink in. I didn't have much trouble letting it sink in, because I still believed that if this is what God wants me to do, then this is what I will do. At the start of mid-term, I asked my parents was there any chance I could go on a break away with my friends somewhere, and Halloween night, James, John, Cormac, Hugh, my cousin Eoin, Uncle Brian, Dad and myself loaded ourselves on to a minibus and set off for a week in London, thanks to my uncles.

Chapter Thirty-Seven

A trip to London. I was delighted to hear Donal express an interest in doing something different. We organised a minibus and headed for Dublin Port, accompanied by his four friends, his cousin Eoin and his uncle Brian. We would meet his other uncles, Kieran and Maurice, once we got to London.

Before we left, I had a talk with Donal's friends in private. He had chosen the four of them to travel with him on this fun trip, but of course his biggest journey lay ahead. In his own inimitable way, he had told them what was going to happen but I wondered if they were fully able to comprehend what it meant.

'We're not doing this lightly,' I said. 'You're going on a journey with Donal and it's terminal. Are you prepared to travel it with him?'

I needed to know if they were strong enough to deal with those final terrible weeks that lay ahead of us. If not, they would be better off acknowledging their difficulties at this stage. No one would blame them or hold it against them. Donal's death was a stark reality and, probably, the first time tragedy would cast its shadow over their young lives. Would they be by his side and share this spiritual experience with him? The lads had no hesitation. They would be with him every step of the way. Prior to this, I suspect, they had seen me as a coach or a tour organiser, a practical man used to being in control. Now they saw me as a father and, listening to me, they were aware that raw grief had to exist alongside the practical necessity of preparing the way for Donal.

So the bags were packed and off we went. Due to flight difficulties, we were driving over and flying home. I was the driver. This was no bad thing, as it forced me to focus on the road and leave my tormented thoughts to one side. We spent the first night in Bewley's Hotel at Newlands Cross, then boarded the ferry the following morning. I watched the lads strolling around the deck, lounging on the chairs, playing the gaming machines, tucking into food. Donal looked no different to any of them. He was full of vigour and laughter. Nothing in his appearance or demeanour suggested that he had only recently received such devastating news.

We arrived in London at around 5 p.m. Maurice had dinner organised for us in a local restaurant, after which we headed for the luxurious four-star Grafton Hotel in the centre of London's shopping district. Donal's sense of style was always sharp. Paul Galvin, the Kerry footballer and fashion aficionado, was his guru and a lot of shopping was planned for the weekend.

The following morning we hit the high street. This was my first experience of shopping with a group of teenagers and I was on a fast learning curve. The merits and demerits of brands like Hollister, Guess, Diesel, Calvin Klein, Homme, G-Star, Levi's and Dockers – to name a few – were scrutinised and discussed with an academic knowledge that was impressive, if incomprehensible to me. Having decided not to make a decision to buy, they then moved on to the next shop, where the process was repeated until everyone agreed to return to the first shop to make their purchase.

Soon they were kitted out to their satisfaction and, laden with carrier bags, we returned to the hotel. I went for a siesta, exhausted from my journey through the fashion thoroughfares of London and the previous day's driving. The lads decided to explore the London Eye but as the queue was too long, they ended up in Trafalgar Square, where they had some fun with the iconic stone lions. I was later informed they were almost arrested. Obviously the London bobbies didn't see the humour of five Irish lads riding on the backs of these magnificent British lions.

On day two, we headed for Thorpe Amusement Park. Donal's prosthesis prevented him taking some of the rides but he availed of everything else. The weekend passed in a blur of shopping, sightseeing and dining out. Donal tasted his first beer and gave it the thumbs down. Then they rather tentatively suggested that they'd like to see what Soho was like or, as they put it, 'the red light district'. Would I be their guide and lead the way? Why not? We wandered around Soho with its neon, glitter and nightclubs. They loved the atmosphere, as well as the belief that they were treading on salacious soil. Two of the braver lads decided to try and enter one of the more exclusive bars. They picked a bar with a female security guard and approached her. Both were over six feet tall, and she stood aside to allow them entry. The lads were so taken aback that they stopped in their tracks.

'You mean you're letting us in?' one of them gasped.

I guess at that point she must have known to look beyond their mature appearance, because she immediately snapped to attention and asked for their identity cards. That was the end of that and we headed back to our hotel, still laughing over the audacity of the lads.

However, Donal and I did have an angry exchange during this trip. I'd been waiting for something to blow up, anticipating his reaction to the shock he'd received when he sat down in front of Michael Capra to hear his fate. He was so intent on being cheerful, yet he was just a sixteen-year-old youth and, despite his bravery, he had not fully taken in the enormity of what he'd been told. He needed to express his anger at the unfairness of it all. And so he did. When he got wind of my private conversation with his friends, he was furious with me for discussing him without his prior knowledge. What I believed had been a protective gesture, he saw as interference. As always, he refused to be singled out for special attention, rejecting labels that would make him different. Independent and spirited, he was determined to control his life until the end. I'd hurt his feelings but I suspected that if he had not had that reason as an excuse, something else would have blown up. His uncle Kieran, after hearing both sides of the argument, acted as an intermediary to help us to understand each other's point of view, but we headed for the airport without resolving our differences.

We were early for our flight and, while the lads explored the shopping malls, Donal and I sat down together to have a heart-to-heart. We talked and cried and talked some more. I'd desperately wanted everything to go well in London, desperately wanted him to forget, just for a short while, all that was to come. As if that was possible. During my student days, I'd studied psychology and philosophy. I knew so much in theory – but what training does a parent have to cope with the impending loss of a precious child? In the end we made up our argument but in the weeks that followed, I saw my son struggle with his anger as he adjusted to the death sentence he'd received. Who else could he vent his frustration on, except his nearest and dearest? I realised he was trying to push me away so that when our parting came, it would not be too painful. As if he could prepare me ... But he was young and inexperienced when it came to understanding the vast reaches of the human heart. His reaction was normal and understandable, a natural stage of grief that he overcame. His innate positivity returned, as did his desire to cram as many experiences as possible into the time left to him.

As a family we had to do a lot of serious talking. We could not avoid the truth or the anguish of such conversations. In one of these discussion with Elma, Donal listed the children he had known and befriended in Crumlin Hospital: those who had fought like him and lost their battle with cancer. His question was no longer, 'Why me?' It had become another, equally unanswerable question: 'Why not me? Why should I be any different to all those other children?' Death was his final referee and Donal had never fought with or questioned a referee's decision in any sport he played. We had to move with him, to try to bring our minds to that profound place where he had found acceptance.

On another occasion, he asked Elma when she was going to return to work after he died. 'I'm going back on the Monday after your funeral,' she told him, knowing that he would expect nothing but the truth from her.

'That's right,' he replied. 'Keep going and don't be sad.' If only it was that easy.

Jema, like us, had to be prepared to let her brother go. She had endured his illness with great fortitude, but her greatest test lay ahead. He asked her to name her first baby boy after him, and she agreed. Such discussions seemed surreal but they were very real. She had to find the strength to laugh with Donal. We all did and, somehow, that was what we did, loudly and often.

The first of the house parties that Donal would organise in the months to come also took place over that period of mid-term. About thirty of his friends came in fancy dress and the house rocked to the boom-boom music he loved. Everyone was having fun. The notion that this was his last Halloween was ludicrous. He danced as hard as anyone, determined to show his friends that he would fight this battle to the bitter end.

He stopped going to school. This was his choice and we supported his decision. He hated the idea of silence falling when he entered a classroom. He didn't want to cause embarrassment to other pupils, who would struggle to find the right words to say to him. What could they say, these young people, when faced with the mortality of one of their own? But he also wanted time to reflect and reach inwardly into the quiet space where his spirituality resided. He stayed at home with Elma, who had given up her job yet again to look after his medical needs. However, he was not forgotten and his teachers were very proactive in creating events that included him.

He accepted an invitation to join his classmates on an outing to the Ardfert Retreat Centre, where a reading of Seamus Heaney's poetry was to be held. To his surprise, the bus passed the expected destination and continued on to Ballyheigue Beach, where various water sport activities had been planned. Unknown to Donal, his mother was in the Ballygarry House Hotel in Tralee, where the owner, Pádraig McGillicuddy, had his helicopter ready to fly her out to meet the lads. I watched them take off, with Elma bravely waving from the back seat, a bottle of holy water in her other hand as the helicopter lifted into the air.

The lads on the beach were surprised to see a helicopter coming in to land so close to them. Things clicked into place when they saw Elma emerge from the rear. Donal and his friends were then given the helicopter ride of their lives. After a few initial swoops and low-level passes, their nervousness disappeared and they began to enjoy the experience.

'Skim the waves,' Donal yelled, egging Pádraig on. 'Go faster, faster, *faster*!'

They were exuberant when they were finally back on terra firma, much to Elma's relief. They had been perfectly safe, Pádraig admitted, but he was carried away by Donal's enthusiasm and enjoyed the experience as much as anyone.

And so the days passed. Donal went regularly with his uncle, Brian to the Kingdom Mart, where Brian is chairman, and enjoyed listening to the rapid-fire auctioneering, the banter and the wit of the farmers. On Friday evenings he'd walk up the road to Brian's house, where they'd eat pizzas and watch a box set or repeats of *Top Gear*, one of Donal's favourite programmes. He also followed the saga of Lance Armstrong with interest. He'd been a fan of the cyclist until the doping stories began to circulate, then lost all interest in him when the truth emerged. To be engrossed by such worldly affairs, to tweet and Facebook, to look forward to the next match, the next concert – it seemed incongruous that these things should occupy his mind, but they did. And yet he was able to talk with the same candour to his friends and to us about his death.

He made us promise we would help him to pass peacefully away at home. No more hospitals. He was not afraid of dying, as long as he could do so in his much-loved and familiar surroundings. It took time to have that conversation without us falling apart but, somehow, in a strange way, having such discussions with him helped us cope. It gave us a sense of purpose, to know that he was depending on us to ease him from one life into the next. He had no doubts in his mind. He was walking into God's arms ... But not just yet. He still had a lot more partying to do. He loved his nights out. The usual teenage curfews went by the wayside and he took full advantage when he managed to secure ID that would admit him and his friends to various nightclubs in Kerry.

We organised a get-together with all his cousins. They met with him and Jema in the Brogue Inn, a familiar landmark for anyone who has driven through Tralee. I looked at this new generation – his Limerick cousins, Carla, Sasha, Ailish, Eadaoin, Richard, Leslie, Rufus and Oisín; his cousins from Kerry, Eoin, Clodagh, Ríos, Riona, and Eoin's girlfriend, Louise; and his Dublin cousins, Amy, James and Christina, who had formed such a bond with him during his time in hospital – and I thought of how much Donal loved hanging out with such exuberant young people. It seemed impossible to imagine that he would not be part of these family gatherings in the future but if that thought crossed his mind, he was not going to let it dominate the enjoyment of the night.

The excursions continued. They included another helicopter ride at the start of an overnight stay in the Riverside Hotel in Tullamore, organised by my brother Kieran's friends. The helicopter quite literally landed outside our front door to collect myself, Donal and his friend John. Compared to me, the two lads were quite relaxed as the chopper lifted above our house and flew over Tralee – after all, they had prior flying experience! Seeing familiar sights from a different perspective was fascinating. By the time we flew over my own home village of Knocklong, I'd forgotten my nervousness as I pointed out the familiar landmarks of my childhood.

We enjoyed our stay in the Riverside Hotel, where we were joined by the rest of Donal's friends and Kieran's sons, Sean and Ronan, and by Elma and Jema, and Jema's friend Vicki. The younger crowd had now swelled to nine and they were intent on enjoying themselves, especially as the hotel had a nightclub, where they danced until the small hours.

As I mentioned earlier, Donal had been determined to learn how to drive and a very patient Brian had succeeded in teaching him. The following morning he was about to have his first experience of driving a Ferrari. After everyone had inspected this magnificent car when Seamus, the owner, pulled up outside the hotel, and the boys in particular had drooled over its classy chassis, Donal sat inside the driver's seat and was given a short lesson by Seamus on how to handle the gears. He was only too delighted to experiment, roaring the engine into life then returning it to a purr. After this short lesson Donal then drove the Ferrari for the first twenty miles of our journey to the village of Adare. Looking back on a video taken at that time, he looks amazingly cool and confident, more like a young man about town in his mid-twenties than a teenager ravaged by cancer. If he'd had his way, he would have enjoyed nothing more than driving the Ferrari all the way to Adare Manor, but he reluctantly relinquished the wheel and the second part of the trip began.

Adare Manor is a luxurious five-star castle hotel located in Adare, one of Ireland's most picturesque villages. We approached Limerick Tunnel in convoy behind the Ferrari but were overtaken by a driver in his 700 cc car. He was determined to overtake each of us in turn. His little car screamed with the effort it took to do this, but the driver had a triumphant look on his face as he passed us by. Hitting the tunnel, however, the Ferrari slipped into the outer lane and roared into life, tearing past everything on its inside, to the shocked dismay of the previously exultant driver. The reverberations of the engine in the tunnel were astonishing and Donal was flushed with excitement by the time we arrived at Adare Manor.

Earlier, he had joked that if he had landed on the grounds of this illustrious castle with its reputation for quality cuisine, he would have strolled in casually and ordered a takeaway burger and chips. The hotel staff, getting wind of his remark, returned the joke and had a burger and chips ready for him on his arrival. For the rest of us it was soup and sandwiches, served in the traditional Adare Manor style. Mary, Donal's grandmother and some of his uncles joined us. For a short time, it was possible to relax and laugh with our family, to reminisce and ease our minds from the reality of our situation.

Such occasions kept us sane and strong as Christmas approached. The spectre of 'an early Christmas' had been avoided, and Donal was able to drive Elma on her shopping expeditions. He was active and involved in all the preparations, determined to enjoy his last Christmas with, as he put it, 'all the trimmings, Mom'.

Chapter Thirty-Eight
Donal's Story

Over the next few weeks at home, a lot of things changed. I dropped out of school to have more time for my life. I was given helicopter rides and a chance to drive a Ferrari, which I took up with no hesitation.

As a family, we went to Lourdes. While I was there, I didn't experience much healing but I went for confession and met a South African priest. I asked him why God could give such an illness to young infants who have not had a life. His reply gave me great comfort: we are not in this life for answers, this life is for lessons and questions – it isn't until heaven that we receive answers.

I met for the first time with my palliative doctor and her team. After that, it kind of hit me that these were the people who were going to help me die. It was like they were fluffing my pillows for a good night's sleep and it sunk in that there was going to be an end soon. That still didn't mean I was going anywhere without a fight.

I had trips to Cork for radiotherapy which would slow the cancer down, but my doctors still warned my parents to have an early Christmas. But because I knew this was going to be my last

Christmas, I still wanted it to be special. Nonetheless, Christmas remained 25 December.

I wanted unique gifts for all the people I loved: signet rings for my four best friends and one that I would wear as well, unique pieces of jewellery for my sister and my mother and other special friends. I didn't ask for any gifts, but somehow my mom managed to bring Santa Claus to the house on Christmas Eve while my friends and cousins were here. He gave a gift to everyone and we had a good laugh.

I got a lot of happiness out of Christmas, we had more house parties and my debs was soon after. I got to bring one of my best friends, Joanne, and went with James and his date for the night.

January came and with it, so did more pain. This led to more radiotherapy and palliative care treatment.

Chapter Thirty-Nine

From October 2012 to March 2013 Donal went to the radiological department in Cork University Hospital for treatment to slow down his cancer. We were also introduced to Dr Patricia Sheahan, Head of the Palliative Care Unit at Kerry General Hospital. She would look after Donal in the final stage of his journey. I'd previously met with one of her palliative care team, and requested that the term 'palliative care' not be used in his presence. Instead, I wanted them to be called the 'pain management' team. I thought I was protecting Donal from terms associated with death. But who was I really protecting? Him or me? Now, looking back, I'm not so sure. I still believe my thinking on this issue was correct, but I really was not ready to face the actuality of those grim words.

I was also anxious about the new medication Donal would receive and was only too conscious of his reaction on the night he'd suffered the seizure in hospital on that previous occasion. I wanted Michael Capra included in the discussions, but Patricia was patient with me throughout our sometimes heated discussions. I'm sure she felt my anger over her intrusion into our son's life, which was now heading into a significant final stage. But she made me aware that it wasn't just Donal who was making this journey. Each one of us was doing so in our own personal way. My anger was part of that grieving process. She had a wealth of experience behind her and, although she permitted me my 'reservations', she was still insistent enough to prescribe the new medication.

Tears were never far away, as I looked at the suffering Donal was enduring and thought of the loss that lay ahead. But I was filled with awe and a bittersweet pride at the way he was coping, at his determination to wring enjoyment from every opportunity that came his way. Christmas was coming and he showed no intention of going anywhere – except into Tralee to shop 'til he dropped. For once, he could buy whatever he liked. Every last penny he received directly from well-wishers was soon spent on presents for his family and friends. He was living on borrowed time, and he was determined to make this Christmas one we would always remember.

'With all the trimmings, Mom', was exactly what Donal enjoyed. Elma heard of a local man who 'did' Santa on Christmas Eve for families. She contacted him and asked if he would visit our house and hand out presents to our family and friends. Santa arranged to call at 5 p.m. on Christmas Eve. Everyone was assembled and waiting. Mary, my mother, was celebrating the day with us, and nearly all Donal's cousins and friends were able to come, as did Santa with a bag full of goodies for everyone. He was a huge hit, especially when it came to handing out the presents. The girls received remote control cuddly toys, while the lads got remote control toys for boys – but they didn't get their gifts unless they sat on Santa's knee for a photograph. There was much laughter and joking when Santa tried to balance six-foot plus boys on his lap as the pictures were taken. He stayed around until well past his allotted time to make sure that we were, indeed, having a merry Christmas.

We attended Midnight Mass. Our prayers came from deep within our souls. For all of us, it was a day of incredibly mixed emotions. We felt joy that Donal had survived to share this special occasion with us and an aching sadness that we would not be together when the feast of Christ's birthday was once again celebrated in our house, twelve months hence.

On St Stephen's night, Donal went out with his friends. They took the bus to Dingle, where the Wren Boy tradition is celebrated with a parade of wren boys in the traditional straw suits or in fancy dress. There was music, song and dance that night and the atmosphere in the town was fantastic. The lads had such a good time that they nearly missed the bus back to Tralee at 3 a.m. It was also the night Donal met Aislinn. They hit it off straight away and a strong friendship developed between them.

Aislinn was going to college but when she was free she would drive to Tralee, and they would go to the cinema together, hang out with friends or visit her house in Ballybunion. She came into Donal's life at a late stage and both were aware that their time together would be short and intense. It really was a special friendship and it upset Donal to know that this relationship would have to end so soon. He had many reasons to live, and

Aislinn became one of them. His cancer was beginning to take its toll on him but he still had more life to grab.

His final rugby match was the Ireland v England Six Nations game, played in February 2013 in the Aviva Stadium. Unfortunately, it was not to be our day and England won. Donal was still active but his bones were becoming increasingly fragile. I watched him anxiously on his way to the exit as he weaved in and out of the heaving crowd. I kept nudging people out of his way, to try and prevent them bumping against him.

One woman, extremely irritated, turned on me. 'Watch what you're doing,' she snapped. 'This is the third time you've pushed against me. Kindly respect other people's space.' I watched Donal moving ahead and quietly told her that my son had terminal cancer. Far from invading her space, I was doing my best to protect him. When I looked back, she was standing in the same position, her face still frozen with shock.

In February Donal was admitted to Marymount Hospice in Cork for observation. His medication was changed and methadone became his base painkilling drug. He had initially rejected going. He knew what a hospice was. He was not about to give up that easily and, to him, a stay in Marymount signalled another stage of his deterioration. Elma and I had to support Dr Patricia and convince him he would benefit greatly from the experience. By now I'd lost my fear of the palliative care unit and had warmed to the professional and compassionate way they worked. Donal eventually agreed to take the ten days in Marymount, where he adjusted to methadone. Our son the druggie, we joked.

During those ten days the palliative team observed his reaction to the new drug. He had to go for radiation treatment to Cork University Hospital each morning. Afterwards he and Elma would browse the shopping centres, take in a film or explore any other diversions the city had to offer. In the hospice, his room was at the end of a corridor. To reach the exit he had to walk past families whose relatives were nearing their natural end. He witnessed many scenes of grief. This added to his awareness of what we would soon endure and so Elma made sure his days were as fully occupied as possible.

While Donal was supposed to be under constant observation, the hospice team accepted that his mother was his best nurse. At this stage the medications were changing on a daily basis, and she had become proficient in his care. He would return for his medication at 6 p.m. each evening and then escape once again to meet up with me or other family members for a meal or a film. Usually, he returned at around 10 p.m. to sleep in the hospice and counted the hours until he could return home to his own bed. He'd objected to staying in the hospice, yet the treatment he received gave him a new lease of life – as we were soon to discover.

Chapter Forty
Donal's Story

They sent me to Marymount Hospice in Cork for ten days while I was being put on methadone as a painkiller. When I came home, it was like I had a new lease of life. My mom organised a weekend trip to Paris with my cousins Eoin, Clodagh, Ríos, Riona and my sister Jema. My mom and uncles came too, we had a good laugh and made nice memories together. When I got home, I was out most weekends with my friends and I had the energy during the week for all the visitors, but I soon began to realise that time was slipping away.

Chapter Forty-One

Magnificent Notre Dame – with its towers and vast transepts, its stunning stained glass windows and grotesque gargoyles – fascinated Donal. According to Elma, who had accompanied him to the cathedral on their trip to Paris, he was mesmerised by the grandeur of this ancient place of worship. As with most Gothic cathedrals, these awesome, soaring spaces are a reminder of our own diminutive presence on this earth and, perhaps, that was what Donal felt when he ceased his explorations and quietly asked his mother, 'Mum, am I really, *really* going to die?'

Elma is brave and forthright, and how could she answer him with anything less than the truth? 'We can only know what the doctors have told us,' she replied. 'But they're not God either, so we don't know when it will happen – or if it will.'

He nodded in acceptance and said, 'Don't worry, Mom. I'm not worried about it. But there's something over here. I must go.' He left her and disappeared behind one of the pillars. Elma believes – and Brian, who was with her and also witnessed his reaction, agrees – that Donal's experience in Notre Dame had a profound spiritual influence on him.

During the trip, he fell and fractured his arm. Despite all Elma's efforts at persuasion, he refused to go to hospital until he returned home. The arm was strapped up to give him some relief, but that was all. Nothing was going to stop him having fun nor would he disappoint his cousins as they visited the usual tourist sights: the Louvre and the Eiffel Tower, the Arc de Triomphe and the Champs-Élysées. Donal had heard about a certain church in Paris where miracles occurred. He didn't know its name or where it was located and, despite everyone's best efforts, it seemed they would have to leave Paris without visiting it. As they were leaving for the airport, however, they discovered where it was. They had time to spare and a decision was made to detour and pay it a visit.

In the Chapel of Our Lady of the Miraculous Medal on Rue du Bac, they attended Mass and Donal recited a prayer of consolation. He loved this church and was reluctant to leave it. As they walked away, they passed a young man begging on the street. Brian stopped to talk to him and discovered he was Irish. The lads immediately wanted to mount a rescue operation and fly him back with them to Ireland. The erstwhile beggar showed no signs of wanting to return home and the lads reluctantly abandoned the idea, when they were reminded by the others that planes don't wait on the tarmac for knights in shining armour. On that note, the Paris trip ended.

But from then on, Elma believed Donal's experience in Notre Dame had changed him in a way she could never describe.

She just knew he had reached a different place, and felt that there was a peace about him from then on, an almost surreal presence. She describes it now as something deeper than acceptance or peace of mind. Whatever happened to him gave him a heightened sense of awareness and his spirituality deepened. He began to feel at ease with himself and his own mortality. He was calm yet focused, taking in everything. He saw things clearly, clearer than we can, even today. Elma would see him looking at something and felt that it wasn't in the same way you or I would see it. It was as if Donal was viewing his world from a different perspective. He started talking much more seriously to his friends. He went down a different road and he was not afraid to die. He told Elma God had him by the hand and he would walk into His arms. This belief was a tremendous comfort to him, and to us. It would have been so much worse if he'd sat in his room crying every day, but he never did.

We were now moving into the spring and a new budding. We kept hoping – maybe … just maybe … Each day was a precious gift and Donal was still active, still striving. He was now meeting a wide circle of people outside his immediate friends. He'd hear of someone who was having difficulties, perhaps drugs or alcohol or some kind of petty crime, something that was going to create problems for them in the future. He would spend time with them and talk about what was going wrong with their lives. Knowing he was going to die gave him the courage to say what needed saying. *Life is precious. Don't squander it.*

He became increasingly upset by the mounting rates of suicide, especially among young people. Some of these took place locally, but there were clusters of such tragedies around the country. I was shocked one evening when I saw a document on his iPod entitled, 'Suicide Letter'. I froze, afraid to open it – yet I knew I must check what he'd written. My heartbeat steadied after reading it but I was on the verge of tears when I asked Elma if she had seen it.

'Yes,' she replied. 'Donal has already shown it to me. He's upset that young people are taking their own lives, while he's been fighting so hard to hold on to his own.'

What upset Donal most was what he saw as the 'glorification' of suicide on social media sites, and a worrying acceptance among some young people that suicide was a 'right', and should be regarded as such. He had written this letter as a response to this attitude. It was not to be published until after his death, he told me, when I asked him about it. He had printed it out and was keeping it upstairs in his bedroom.

Unknown to us, outside events were moving into place and this letter was to have a profound effect, not only on Donal's life but also on us, his parents.

Shortly after this, we received word that one of Donal's teachers, Ruairí O'Rahilly, had nominated him for the Radio Kerry/*Kerry's Eye* Local Hero Award. This award celebrates those who have made a difference to their community and to other people's lives. Ruairi cited the fundraising Donal had undertaken for Crumlin Hospital and the original story he wrote about his cancer that had been published in his school magazine.

Donal won the award. It was a unanimous decision by the judging panel, who had been inundated with nominations from all over the county. 'Donal Walsh is a unique and inspirational young man,' said Chief Superintendent Pat Sullivan, who chaired the panel. 'I've known Donal and his story for some time, and his courage and dignity have never ceased to move me. Much of An Garda Síochána's resources and efforts are focused on our youth: after all, they are tomorrow's adult society. People like Donal make our job so much easier, because his leadership qualities and fundraising efforts are inspirational to all his peers. Above all, the example Donal continues to set through his courageous fight in the face of the most difficult personal circumstances is what all of us aspire to. Quite simply, it is of heroic proportions.'

Donal, being Donal, shrugged off such praise but we could see he was delighted to receive this recognition. The award was presented to him at home with a small media presence. One of the journalists, who had read his essay, asked if he had other writings. Donal shook his head but Elma, aware of the 'suicide letter', asked him to show it. Initially, he refused. He had his own plan for the letter and it was only after much persuasion from Elma, who had a way of coaxing him to do her bidding, that he went upstairs to get it. She recognised its importance and felt that the impact of his message would be stronger if the letter was published while he was still alive. But even she had no idea what she was unleashing when Donal reluctantly handed it over.

I've had experience over the years of dealing with the media and I immediately noticed the reaction of the journalists who read it. What Donal had written touched a raw nerve. Something that was different than the financial collapse of the economy and the unrelenting spewing of bad news. A message from a dying boy, asking young people to value their most precious possession. Life.

The previous September, after a particularly harrowing day in his courtroom in Killarney, Terence Casey, the South Kerry Coroner, had spoken publicly about the issue of suicide in the county. Of the eight deaths inquired into in that sitting, six were due to suicide. All the victims were males, aged from fourteen to fifty-eight. 'Those who take their own lives don't take into consideration the hurt, sorrow and pain that they leave behind them,' he'd said to the family and friends of the deceased at the close of the proceedings. In his ten years as coroner, he had never seen so many suicides in one sitting. Help was available but suicidal people did not know where to look for this help, he added.

He was one of many voices speaking out about this problem, but now, with Donal, this was the first time that a sixteen-year-old youth, desperate to cling onto life, had made that same appeal. His was a stark but positive message, delivered in unflinching terms and no one – no matter how hard-boiled and cynical – could doubt its truth or sincerity.

Donal's letter and essay, along with coverage of the Local Hero Award, made the front page of *Kerry's Eye*, and received further publicity when the front page went online. After that, there was no holding back the tide of publicity. Our lives were about to be turned upside down once again – but in a way we'd never anticipated.

Chapter Forty-Two
Donal's 'Suicide Letter'

A few months left, he said. There it was: I was given a timeline on the rest of my life. No choice, no say, no matter. It was given to me as easy as dinner.

I couldn't believe it – that all I had was sixteen years here, and soon I began to pay attention to every detail that was going on in this town.

I realised that I was fighting for my life for the third time in four years, and this time I have no hope. Yet still I hear of young people committing suicide and I'm sorry, but it makes me feel nothing but anger.

I feel angry that these people choose to take their lives, to ruin their families and to leave behind a mess that no one can clean up.

Yet I am here with no choice, trying as best I can to prepare my family and friends for what's about to come, and leave as little a mess as possible.

I know that most of these people could be going through financial despair and have other problems in life, but I am at the depths of despair and, believe me, there is a long way to go before you get to where I am.

For these people, no matter how bad life gets, there are no reasons bad enough to make them do this: if they slept on it or looked for help, they could find a solution, and they need to think of the consequences of what they are about to do.

So please, as a sixteen-year-old who has no say in his death sentence, who has no choice in the pain he is about to cause and who would take any chance at even a few more months on this planet, appreciate what you have, know that there are always other options and help is always there.

Chapter Forty-Three

Initially, the publicity that followed the publication of the letter angered Donal. As the recipient of the Local Hero Award, he'd expected some local publicity and, instead, he was suddenly being presented as a voice for suicide prevention. It took a few days before he realised that in fact his message was very important and that he was in a unique position to ask young people to focus on the valuing of life, not its destruction. This simple request was made all the more powerful by the fact that he had such a short time within which to deliver it.

South Kerry Coroner Terence Casey quickly rowed in behind Donal and agreed that the suicide rate and the glorification of the act of suicide among young people were wrong. This statement from such an eminent commentator drew the attention of the national media. Soon, every radio and television station wanted to talk to Donal. It was clear that we had to make some very considered decisions. Our son was too ill to be subjected to the rigours of the media. They were only doing their job but we, as Donal's parents, also had to do *our* job. We didn't want our remaining time with him to be spun out in the media spotlight, and so we were careful in selecting who would interview him.

We consulted at length with Patricia Sheahan and Michael Capra on the wisdom of Donal accepting an invitation to appear on *The Saturday Night Show*. Finally, it was agreed that this particular show, because of its younger audience profile, was the right medium for him. The presenter, Brendan O'Connor, is a plain-talking interviewer and we believed he would not exploit Donal in any way during the interview. Fortunately, we were justified in our belief.

Elma travelled to Dublin with Donal, and they met Brendan on the Friday evening at their hotel. Brendan spent two hours building up trust with Donal, who, initially, was quiet when they met and a little overcome by the occasion. Brendan later told us he feared the medication Donal was taking would affect him during the interview, but Donal soon relaxed. He'd just started using a wheelchair after much protesting on his part, but Brendan was anxious that he should walk onto the set. Donal was equally determined to do so, although he was growing weaker and a fall, no matter how slight, could break another bone.

The wheelchair had been strenuously resisted when it was first delivered to our house. It was outside in the driveway when his friends arrived to inspect it. They began to play with it. They raced Donal up and down the path, whizzed along the road. If he could have managed it, he would have done a wheelie. They all took turns experimenting with it and ended up breaking it. I suspect Donal hoped that that was the end of it, but it was essential for his own safety. By the time the replacement was delivered, his mindset had changed. It had become a fun toy to his friends and, as such, it was acceptable and he was prepared to use it.

He was in the wheelchair when he arrived at the RTÉ studios on the Saturday night. None of us had any idea what to expect, and we were astonished to find photographers waiting for us and a film crew filming the proceedings. Brendan was protective and easy with Donal. I suspected he too was a little nervous. This was an important interview, probably one of the most important he would ever do, and he was dealing with someone whose grasp on life was very slender. It was Donal's first time speaking to such a wide audience, and I hoped he would be able to get through the interview without faltering. I'd no doubt he would give it his usual 100 per cent, but would that be enough this time? His adrenaline was flowing however and, as had happened so often in the past, when he was presented with a challenge, he was determined to grasp it.

His medical supports, Michael and Patricia, had also prepared for this event. Ambulances were on standby, teams were in place in Tralee, Dublin Airport and Crumlin Hospital to assist Donal if his condition worsened during the two days he was in Dublin. But he was high on excitement and that energy kept him going. He practised walking on stage and felt satisfied that he could do it with confidence when the cameras were rolling. I won't recount the interview word by word. It was well constructed and is freely available on YouTube. He was the first interviewee on that evening's show. All his nervousness left him when he walked onto that set. It seemed as if a light was switched on inside him. He spoke with conviction and answered Brendan's questions unflinchingly.

'They gave me a few months, but I've been here longer than a few months,' he said, and added that he was not prepared to take deadlines on board.

As I listened to him, I thought it was ironic that he looked so healthy. Apart from a sling supporting his arm from the fall in Paris, he could have been any normal young man discussing any other subject but death. I thought of all the times I'd seen him laid so low that it was impossible to imagine him ever rising from his bed. Yet then, we still had hope. We believed tomorrow would come and come again. We'd travelled so far since that August weekend when Donal, unable to play any longer for the 'Naries', had complained of a pain in his knee and limped dolefully off the pitch. *The Saturday Night Show* was proving to be an emotional rollercoaster for all of us.

Brendan talked him through his illness to date and the prognosis. He then mentioned the well-known Irish writer, Nuala O'Faolain, who, on being diagnosed with terminal cancer, admitted in a famous radio interview that the light had gone from her life.

'I wouldn't look at it that way at all,' Donal said. 'All I see are the good supports I'm getting in life ... Obviously, I'm not looking forward to dying. But I'm not thinking about that. If there's anything negative, it's about all the beautiful things I'm leaving behind.' He went on to speak about Jema, and how much it hurt him that he would not be around to see her being happy and successful in her life, and his friends also.

Jema, Elma and I sat in the front row of the audience and tried to control our feelings, especially when the camera zoomed in on us. When Brendan asked me how I felt about my son I said, 'He's a giant.' I found it hard to speak. The emotions welling inside the three of us were almost impossible to control. But the eyes of the nation were on us. If Donal could be so composed, then we had to cope with our overwhelming sadness in private.

'I should be where he is,' Elma said when Brendan spoke to her and I silently echoed her words.

Brendan had warned Donal that his questions would be blunt, but that was not a problem for him. 'You've come to terms with – or made peace with – the fact that you're going to die?' Brendan said.

Would our son hesitate and be unable to face this very emotional question? I need not have worried. Donal replied that he'd have to deal with it eventually and added, 'I wasn't going to spend my time at home moaning about it ... "Oh! It's coming soon, it's coming soon." I might as well get on with my life and make the most of it. There's no point in me sitting around, crying about what I'm leaving behind, when I can appreciate it while I'm here.'

Brendan asked Donal about the fundraising he had done for Crumlin Hospital and, in particular, for St John's Ward.

'It's been in an awful state for the last four years,' Donal admitted. 'It was built in 1970 with one-family bedrooms. So you could have a parent with a child, and maybe a brother or sister, who would sleep on the floor beside them.' He described the furnishings as a wardrobe and sink and how, by the time he arrived there as a patient in 2008, two families were being squashed into the one room. The audience listened in shock, as Donal related the difficulties that staff endured in Crumlin as they carried out their life-saving duties. The only overt reaction among those listening was a startled exclamation from Brendan when Donal mentioned the bathroom facilities.

'There's one bathroom between eighteen kids,' he said. 'The conditions are a disgrace in the ward. Last June they started renovating and, hopefully, they are nearly done. But I can't say enough for the staff,' he added. 'It's unreal. Once you go in there, the nurses become like a second mom.'

Donal's comments were a grim reminder of the reality that patients and their families have to endure as they struggle through the most difficult period of their lives. Two years before he was born, that was when the promises to build a national children's hospital began. We'd listened to discussion after discussion on this subject, but our son was now going to die before the first sod was turned.

Brendan then asked Donal about his faith and how important it was to him.

'It's a huge part of me,' he replied. 'I wouldn't be where I am at all without it. I see God as giving me this challenge.' This led Brendan to question him about the issue of youth suicide and the letter that had led us to this moment.

'I didn't want them to see suicide as a solution to any of life's problems,' said Donal. 'It hurts me to see them think about it, to see it among their friends. It kills me because I'm here, fighting for my life for the third time. I've no say in anything and I'm still here, waking up every day. They think they have a problem and this might be a solution. That does make me angry. I'm not going to lie about it.' He went on to say that suicide had become more acceptable in society and added, 'I wouldn't want people to ever see this as a permanent solution to a temporary problem. If I'm meant to be a symbol for people to appreciate life – not just suicide, but life more in general – then I'm happy to die if that's what I'm dying for.'

Brendan ended the interview by asking him if there were any other ambitions he would like to fulfil, or things he would like to do before he died, to which Donal replied, 'Obviously, if I'd had the time, I'd have travelled the world ... New Zealand, bungee jumping – all those things. But I won't get to see that in life now, so as long as I find peace over the next few weeks, I'm content in my life. And I'll be happy enough.'

Donal's interview lasted for nineteen minutes and eleven seconds. In that time there were no texts, tweets, Facebook notifications. Nothing but silence. Donal had not only silenced the studio audience, but also the viewers throughout the country.

But all that changed after the interview. Brendan and Donal had worked well together. They'd sparked off each other, the perfect interviewer and interviewee. The excitement in the green room was palpable when we retired there. All hell was breaking loose on the various social media forums, including Twitter, where Donal was trending. His interview had gone viral. His Twitter account registered a jump from a couple of hundred followers to many thousands within minutes, not just in Ireland but globally.

I was new to Twitter and unsure of what was happening. 'What does 'trending' mean?' I asked Jema.

'It means he's the hottest thing on Twitter,' she replied and explained how the process worked. At a later point, she admitted, 'It's okay to explain what "trending" means to a few people, but when the phone calls keep coming and you've explained it fifty times, it does get a bit tiresome.' But she, like us, found the whole experience a welcome distraction. It offered us a brief respite from all that awaited us when we returned home.

The following day, as Elma wheeled Donal along Merrion Street, a jeep pulled in beside us and a woman jumped out. She ran straight to him and hugged him, and thanked him for his interview. Donal had no sooner recovered from the shock of this encounter when another woman stopped to compliment him on the show. And so it continued as Elma wheeled him around St Stephen's Green, with strangers stopping every few minutes to talk to him. On the evening before the interview, when Elma brought him to the Dundrum Town Centre for a meal, he had simply been an anonymous boy in a wheelchair. Now he was instantly recognisable and he was rather thrilled by this sudden rise to fame. But he was also anxious to be back home, where his friends were waiting, excited and thrilled for him. They never faltered in their promise to support him through every stage of his final journey. But I will let their collective voices now tell their own story ...

Chapter Forty-Four
James, John, Cormac and Hugh

He looked great on television on *The Saturday Night Show*, and he was texting us from the green room, having a laugh because he was trending on Twitter. But it was also important to him that he was able to say what he did. It was the 'Suicide Letter' that started it all and it was never meant to happen. He didn't want it published until after his death, in case people thought he was a know-it-all, showing off and just trying to draw attention to his own situation.

There'd been a lot of suicides – we knew personally of three young people who'd taken their lives – and that's when he wrote the letter. He was fighting for every minute he could live. He didn't want deadlines on his life, and it made him sad that there were others who didn't feel their lives were worth fighting for.

Donal rarely talked about the sad stuff, the cancer. But then, sometimes, we'd have conversations so deep, you'd never think sixteen- or seventeen-year-olds would talk about the things we did. We'd just be together, the five of us in his bedroom, and he'd talk about his funeral or the way he was fighting to hold on to every extra minute. He told us we had to do the very best we could with our lives. He'd be lying on his bed and he'd say, 'This is it, lads. You need to express everything that's on your mind, because I'll be gone and then it'll be too late.'

But we didn't process that in our minds. We'd start fighting with him and saying, 'No, you're not going anywhere,' and he'd say, 'All right, then,' and we'd talk about something else. You're not meant to die at sixteen. Or to hear your best friend talking about dying, like it was something natural and not frightening. So we didn't really believe he was going to die. He'd beaten the cancer twice and we reckoned he could beat it again, especially as he looked so well. And he wouldn't give in. It didn't matter that his breathing was bad or he'd be in loads of pain when he was walking. He still wanted to go down the town and see what was going on. He never wanted anyone to think he was sick.

He'd say, 'Come on, lads, let's go up the town and have a laugh.' He was still the same Donal, even when he was told to have an early Christmas. But he didn't die before Christmas. Instead, he gave us rings with our initials on them as presents. We'd our suspicions, as he kept asking us about our finger sizes and then he rang and said, 'Come on over, lads. I've something to give you.'

That was before the big Christmas party, when everyone was there with Santa and the presents. This was just us and there was nothing emotional about it. He said, 'It's just something to remember me by,' and gave the rings to each of us. We wear them all the time now and they'll help us remember what he taught us.

You never know what's going to happen in the future. Life can throw all sorts of things at us. Some of them are small and they seem big at the time. But Donal's cancer really was as big as it gets. And, yet, in the middle of it all, he showed us how important it is to stay positive through all our problems.

We've great memories of all the things we got to do before he died. Like the fun we had in London, with Fionnbar leading us down through Soho and all the house parties Donal organised. We had the first party a few days after we came back from London. That was Halloween and it was a fancy dress party. We'd another three after that. They were all held in Donal's house, with a proper DJ set up and the lights flashing and the rooms packed with all our friends. There'd be a great atmosphere – and Donal would be in the middle of it all, having a brilliant time.

When Make-A-Wish built the den for him, we used to hang out there for a few years. But when his chest got bad, it was too cold so we used to chill out in his bedroom. We'd plan all the things we'd do with him. Like skydiving – he wanted to try that before he died but it didn't happen – and crazy stuff, like swimming the canal or running naked through Manor West. But we were too lazy and too busy, watching movies or talking about school stuff, or sport, girls too, and music. And then, sometimes, the sad stuff.

The first time he was diagnosed with cancer, you'd think he'd be angry, but he got past that and just focused on getting better.

And that's what happened the second time too. But the third time … you'd imagine he'd crack then and stay in his room, crying his eyes out, but he told us that maybe it was God's plan. One of us had to be the first to die and, if his dying made a difference to someone else who felt their life wasn't worth living, then he was happy to sacrifice his own. That was how far his thinking had come. We thought it was amazing that a sixteen-year-old could reason it out like that.

When Donal got word that his cancer was terminal, we called over to see him. We knew something was wrong but there were some other people in the house, and he was laughing and talking like everything was normal. So, we figured things had gone okay with his shoulder. Then everyone left and there were just the five of us in his bedroom. We asked him what was wrong. Was the news bad or good, or what? He'd put on the saddest song in the world, 'Nine Crimes' by Damien Rice, and then he told us the truth. We all started bawling crying. We couldn't help it, and he was laughing at us, crying like babies, like it was all a joke and he'd tell us to wise up and get real. But he wasn't joking. It was true and this was his way of dealing with it, I guess – being told he should have an early Christmas.

There are lots of memories, but one that will always stay with us is when the lights would be off and we'd be chilled out on his bed. There'd be a movie on and Elma would come up with popcorn and stuff, and it all seemed so normal, as if things would never change.

He was getting a lot of publicity by then, all the fundraising and the Local Hero Award, and it really took off after he was on television. People were calling him 'an inspiration'. He used to get angry at that, because that wasn't how he saw it at all. He'd say, 'It's what any of you'd do if you were in my place.'

When we were alone with him, we'd say, 'But that's what you are, Donal. It's actually incredible what you're doing by staying so strong.' He didn't want to know any of that. He just wanted people to listen to what he had to say about life being precious.

The last thing he always said to us was, 'I'll see you tomorrow, lads', so there was never going to be a final goodbye.

Chapter Forty-Five

Letters started to arrive almost immediately after Donal's appearance on *The Saturday Night Show*. Thousands of letters from people of all ages, along with the constant flow of support through email, Twitter and Facebook. The letters that delighted Donal most were the ones he received from schools, particularly from the female pupils who thought he was inspirational but still 'a ride'! The boys were more restrained. They called him a 'legend' and an 'inspiration', and we were delighted that he was able to enjoy such recognition from his peers.

One seventy-five-year-old man told us how he'd carried the burden of his brother's suicide for fifty years. After Donal's interview, he was finally able to let go and appreciate that the guilt he carried was the mess his brother had left behind. A mother told how her seventeen-year-old son had broken down in tears after the programme, and admitted that he'd attempted suicide some weeks previously. He was now receiving therapy and his mother thanked Donal for saving his life.

But his words disturbed some who heard them. Those who

wrote to newspapers or argued online that his message was 'an over-simplification' of the tragedy of suicide. Accusations were made, that he was judging those who battle with depression and succumb to suicide. Nothing could be further from the truth. Donal was using the language of a sixteen-year-old when he wrote: 'I feel angry that these people choose to take their lives, to ruin their families and to leave behind a mess that no one can clean up.' His language was direct but not judgemental. The manner in which he accepted his illness and his dignity in the face of his untimely death gave him the moral authority to speak out. His words opened up a highly charged debate on the challenges surrounding youth suicide.

Donal's days were numbered, but he still had work to do to spread his message.

Brendan from *The Saturday Night Show* had asked him to bring his original school essay up to date. He also asked Donal's permission to publish the letter he had written about suicide. Throughout the following week, Donal dictated to Elma a final section for the essay – on his illness and its destructive path. He'd also been working on a piece he called 'Climbing God's Mountain'. This was a spiritual essay that helped him to understand the purpose of his short life. The three pieces were emailed to Brendan, who planned to have them published in the *Sunday Independent.*

Brendan had some difficulty fitting all three pieces on the two allocated pages of the paper. The editorial staff discussed how they could be cut, but when Brendan asked which piece should be left out, they found it impossible to decide. In the end, Donal's writings were published verbatim, and he had the thrill of being paid for his first published work. He could now describe himself as a writer, in the best Kerry tradition.

Shortly afterwards, we received a letter from the editor of a rival newspaper, who wrote: 'In normal life he would be offered the position of a resident feature journalist with any international newspaper and they would be privileged to have him!'

When I opened the newspaper and saw Donal's words in print, I was once again filled with amazement, especially when I read 'Climbing God's Mountain'. I wondered how he could attain such clarity of thought when he knew the enormity of what he had to face. Yet he was still able to concentrate his mind and write these words, in the hope that they would encourage others to appreciate what they had, even in their darkest, most despairing days.

Chapter Forty-Six
I've grown fully in both body and mind by climbing God's mountains

I live in a part of the world that is surrounded by mountains. I can't turn my head without finding a bloody hill or mountain and I suppose those were God's plans for me. To have me grow up around mountains and grow climbing a few too. And that's exactly what I've done, I may have grown up in body around them but I've fully grown and matured in mind climbing His mountains.

He's had me fight cancer three times, face countless deaths and losses in my life; He's had my childhood dreams taken off me – but at the end of the day, He's made me a man.

I am always called brave, heroic, kind, genuine, honourable and so many other kind compliments, but I have to try and explain to everyone why I seem to reject them. I have never fought for anyone but myself, therefore I cannot be brave or heroic; I've only been kind because my religion has taught me so. What impact could I ever make on the world if I was fake, or how could I ever be honourable if I was not honoured to be here?

DONAL'S MOUNTAIN

I am me. There is no other way of putting it, little old Donal Walsh from Tralee: one body, one mind with a few other cobwebs and tales thrown in.

I've climbed God's mountains, faced many struggles for my life and dealt with so much loss. And, as much as I'd love to go around to every fool on this planet and open their eyes to the mountains that surround them in life, I can't. But maybe if I shout from mine, they'll pay attention.

If I start to accept these compliments, I'm afraid of what I'll become. Will I be braver than YE? Will I be kinder than YE? More genuine than YE? Or more honourable than YE? Better than YE? No. I can never accept that there is a YE. We are all the same: we are all given one body, one mind. The only difference for me is that I'm looking from the mountain.

Chapter Forty-Seven

Donal's condition was deteriorating daily. He was sleeping longer and waking later in the day. He was asleep one day, when the President's secretary rang to advise us that President Michael D. Higgins wished to speak to him. I took the call and listened, as the President expressed his feelings about the interview. He was proud of Donal, impressed by his courage and honesty, and by the message of encouragement he was sending out to young people in distress. He spoke to Elma a while longer and promised to call back when Donal was awake. True to his word, the President phoned back later – the first of a number of calls Donal was to receive from him over the following weeks.

Regrettably, we were forced to turn down an invitation to visit him in Áras an Uachtaráin. Donal was too ill to attempt the journey to the presidential residence in the Phoenix Park, much to his disappointment – and the disappointment of Jema and his friends, who'd also been invited. I'm sure President Higgins, whose rapport with young people is well known, was also regretful that this meeting could not take place, but he continued to stay in touch. No matter how weak he was, Donal would rise from his bed to take the call. Each time they said goodbye, I wondered if this would be their last conversation.

Despite his failing health, Donal still remained mentally active and engaged. Directly after the Brendan O'Connor interview, Kathleen Lynch, Minister of State for Disability, Equality and Mental Health, phoned me. She asked if Donal could do one further interview that would re-emphasise his message to live life and not take suicide as an option. Initially, I was unaware of her identity when I took the call. Donal was resting and, as I needed to discuss her request with him and Elma, I asked her to phone back the following day. When she heard the name, Elma quickly filled me in on who this lady was and her ministerial position.

When Minister Lynch phoned back, I apologised for not recognising her name, but that was the least of her worries. She admitted that when the discussion took place among her colleagues as to who would be the most appropriate person to call the father of a dying child, she decided that if anyone was going to make this difficult request, it should be her.

We spoke to Donal about doing the interview. When he agreed, Minister Lynch put us in contact with Gerry Raleigh, Head of Suicide Prevention with the Health Service Executive. We asked that the interview be conducted by Jerry O'Sullivan from Radio Kerry. He was the original interviewer for the Local Hero Award. Donal was familiar with him and did not need the added stress of dealing with a stranger. This was all agreed, and both Jerry and Gerry Raleigh came to our house to work with Donal on how his message should be presented.

What Donal had to say could not be couched in diplomatic language, and so there was a certain amount of negotiation with the HSE as to how it should be worded. We had to do a number of takes. I was anxious that Donal would not be exhausted by the cameras and the activity taking place around him. He refused to use his oxygen tank – by then, he was depending on it to help him breathe – but he wanted to come across as vibrantly as he did on Brendan's show. By the seventh take, I was afraid his message was being lost in an effort to make it less controversial. I declared that I would request all tapes and refuse to allow publication unless his message was clear and unambiguous. I believe that words can become too sanitised around this catastrophic and, often, impulsive decision.

On Brendan's show he'd used words that may have offended some people. He spoke about the 'mess' people leave behind when they end their lives. But Donal was appealing directly to young people contemplating suicide and, in the direct language of a sixteen-year-old, pleading with them to ask for help. He wanted them to believe in their future, to look forward – as he was unable to do – and to give life a second chance.

I was calmed down by Gerry and Elma, but I was still adamant that Donal's meaning should be clearly understood. In all, it took eleven takes before everyone was satisfied.

The difference in Donal's appearance between his television interview with Brendan and now, on this occasion, was obvious. He was unhappy with how he looked when he saw the final take. It brought home to him the difference those few days had made since that memorable night on *The Saturday Night Show*. The medication was taking its toll on him now too, as well as his cancer. His breathing was laboured, he looked frail and it was clear he was very ill. Yet he still found the strength to do those numerous takes and speak openly to his peers.

'This will have more effect!' we told him, when he talked about how ill he looked – but he was not consoled. We were telling the truth. His appearance added a more immediate and powerful impact to his message. His desire to cling to life, no matter how hard he had to fight for those extra weeks, spoke louder than any words.

Chapter Forty-Eight
Donal's Message on the
HSE Suicide Prevention Website

No one is going to judge you at all. Everyone has to open up. It's something everyone has to do. Why keep it to yourself, when people you love, and that love you, are there to help you? They want to help you. They want to get rid of those feelings you're feeling.

When I'm feeling low because of what happened to me, I'll always take time to think. I'll try to realise where the good is in my life over the bad things that make me feel low. I'd talk to my parents. Or I'd usually find a friend to talk to. And we'd look ahead in life. We'd see where I was going to go, what I was going to do. We'd talk a lot about what my dreams and hopes are for the future. They never stop at the present or the past.

So, I'd say to someone who is standing in a room ... I remember when I feel that there are no windows or doors – just black ... Take time and a door will open. Someone will be at that door. And you will go to the door as well.

Anyone can find a window. But they first have to ask and it takes a lot of courage, as well, to ask – and to search for their door.

Chapter Forty-Nine

Back at home again, the postman continued to call. The daily reading of selected letters gave Donal tremendous consolation. I use the word 'selected' deliberately. While most letters were supportive, especially those from families that had encountered suicide, some promised 'miracle cures' from various plant extracts or other natural sources. We had no wish to censor his correspondence but, by now, the tumours were becoming visible in his bone structure.

Cancer does not only attack the individual, it also affects everyone within its environment. It makes you ask why God could allow this to happen to your family. You pray for a miracle and look up every possible cure. At different stages along Donal's journey, we went down all these paths and investigated each possibility that came our way. Some cures were very dubious and cost a great deal of money. They made us question the motivation of people offering them – both from a 'medicinal' and a 'faith' point of view. We were at our most vulnerable, and it shocked us that some people sought to gain financially from us when our lives were in crisis. We investigated most of these options and knew they would have no effect, but still they continued to be presented to us. The battle was lost and cures that came with the advice, 'Why not try it? It might cure you and it certainly won't harm you', had to be ignored, no matter how well-meaning the intention of the sender might be. We could not ask a teenager with only weeks to live to start a diet of powders and extracts that were mostly vile to taste. Looking back over those years, when we still believed hope was possible, I can say with conviction that those who offer 'miracle cures' are genuine only when the offer comes free and without conditions.

One unusual but sincere 'cure' was offered to us by a friend who was working on seaweed extracts. There had been some good results with his products in the area of bovine health, and he came to the house with a very strange offer. He knew there was a million-to-one chance that the cure would work – it had never been tried on humans – but he said he would always regret not coming to us if, at some future date, this treatment was discovered to have curative results for cancer sufferers. To alleviate our fears, he offered to be the first to take the supplement, to prove there were no side effects. We agreed that Donal, myself and our friend would take it on a trial basis. For the following month we took the same extract daily. The only beneficial effect my friend and I experienced however was the incredible regularity of our bowel movements on a daily basis. It did no harm but, sadly, it also did not slow the growth of Donal's tumours.

Another cure promised benefits from the aloe vera plant. The plant had to be five years old; the leaves picked at night after three days without rain, chopped up in the dark, and stored in darkness in a fridge. If you have ever seen the aloe vera plant, you'll know it's quite thorny. The idea of cutting the leaves in the dead of night and being lacerated by the thorns was not a particularly appealing option.

'It might cure my cancer,' mused Donal when he studied the instructions. 'But sure, I'd have no fingers left by the time I'd cut it up in the dark.' Right to the end, his sense of humour never failed him.

For those last few weeks Donal resisted death every step of the way. The oxygen machines were used as little as possible. He wanted to climb the stairs each day and reach his own room by himself. I was determined to carry him up the stairs if necessary, so that he would reach his bed without this superhuman effort. This became less of a possibility however as the tumours grew. His bones were now too brittle, and I would probably have broken them if I'd attempted to lift him in my arms.

As I watched him look up from his wheelchair to the fifteen steps that would bring him upstairs, I began to understand what was on his mind when he wrote 'Climbing God's Mountain'. This was the final mountain he had to climb. It was taking him about ten to fifteen minutes to reach the top step. But he needed to prove to himself that he wasn't giving up. It was agony to watch him struggle up the stairs. There had to be an easier way.

At his check-up the following day, Patricia agreed that a chairlift would help with his palliative care. We contacted the firm responsible for installing them and asked how quickly this could be done. Initially, we were told it would take about four days to complete. A man agreed to call and take the measurements, but when he arrived and saw Donal, he took in the situation at a glance. About an hour later he called back with a solution. He had planned to install a chairlift in a convent the following day but as Donal's need was more immediate, we would receive it instead. He also told us to call him when we needed the chairlift removed. He would be with us within an hour, he promised. We accepted his thoughtful offer. The kindness of strangers was a river that never stopped flowing. But we had no desire to ever have to make that particular call. Hours were becoming precious, as we held on to Donal and he held onto life. He had survived Christmas, Easter, and on May Day he turned to Elma and said, 'Hey, Mom, I made summer!'

We knew we were coming close to the end. Tumours were appearing all over his body, yet he still got up every day and spent time either with his friends or going for a drive to Fenit or Ballyheigue with Elma. On the shore he watched the vastness of the natural beauty he was leaving behind. Every single day some of his friends called, as did his Kerry cousins, including the younger boys, Jack and Darragh. They filled the house with their energy, their music, their laughter. And still the letters, heartbreaking and heartwarming, fell through the letterbox every morning. Representatives from different religious denominations wrote to tell him that in churches, temples and mosques, they were using his interview as material for their various sermons. He was astonished by this outpouring, and heartened by the support that came from across the country.

He was now sleeping for a good part of the day. He arose around 4 p.m. and spent time on Facebook, where, to his delight, he now had twenty thousand 'likes'. His followers on Twitter continued to increase in number and he remained an avid tweeter.

An overnight nurse was organised but her presence was only needed for two nights. This was still a tremendous relief, as it gave Elma a chance to sleep for a few hours and recover some energy for the day ahead. This nurse did not intrude on our lives and did not disturb Donal unless he called for assistance. How difficult it must be for these people to do their jobs, especially when they are nursing a terminally ill patient of such tender years. The chairlift was also not needed for very long. On Friday, 10 May, Donal stayed up with his friends for only a few hours. They came by at 6 p.m. and by 9 p.m. he texted us to say that he needed them to leave. I dropped them home and promised to keep them up to date on how he was.

When I returned, Donal had retired to bed, with the night nurse in attendance. Earlier that evening, we'd suspected his health was deteriorating very rapidly. It was a subtle shift, yet we were acutely conscious of every change in his condition. During the early part of the night he took a turn for the worse and became extremely uncomfortable. We were called regularly to assist in getting him up to the bathroom or to try and settle him into a comfortable position. The night nurse phoned Patricia, who arrived and medicated him in an effort to give him some rest. It was a long night, impossible to sleep for any length of time.

The following morning Donal's medication was increased. By 11 a.m. the change in his condition was more apparent. I asked Patricia if it was time for us to call the priest, and she agreed. First Communions were taking place in the parish and it was difficult for the priests who had been so close to Donal to come immediately. Fr Pádraig Walsh from the adjoining parish was free.

He was at our door within minutes. We talked in the kitchen, while Elma prepared Donal for his visit. This was it. The beginning of the end. My mind raged against it but when I escorted Fr Pádraig to Donal's room, I listened to his quiet voice reciting the prayers for the sick and bestowing a final blessing on our son, with great gentleness and with deep compassion. We were all moved by the ceremony and drew strength from the power of those final prayers. At this point Jema, Brian, Elma and I were the only family members in the house.

'Father, what is it like on the other side?' Donal asked when the praying ended.

'I'm not sure, Donal. But wherever you are going will be a much better place, because you are there,' Pádraig replied. 'Are you afraid?'

'No, Father, just a little nervous,' our son replied. He had to find the strength to let go our hands and enter the final stage of his life's journey but he was 'just a little nervous'!

How we wished we could hold his hands forever. Without hesitation, Elma and I would have given our own lives to see him returned to full health. But that was not in the Divine Plan. As the South African priest in Lourdes had said to him, 'We are not in this life for answers; this life is for lessons and questions – it isn't until heaven that we receive answers.'

We began calling our family. They knew by our voices that it was time for them to come. One by one they arrived and for the remainder of the day, our house was like central station. Food appeared on the table as if by miraculous intervention, laden plates of sandwiches, scones and cakes. Tea was brewed, coffee poured. This was a gathering of our family, like so many in the past, and their support helped us to stay upright. To keep going, as Donal expected us to do. At one point a group of us had gathered in Donal's room. He had been sleeping but when he stirred and looked around, he groaned, 'Hi, I'm going feckin' nowhere today!'

We laughed. Black humour is always appreciated and our son had become a master at it. But our talking was disturbing him, so we cleared everyone from the room and sat with him in shifts. He was never left alone. At one stage when I was there with Brian and Brendan, his twin uncles, the three of us standing at the end of his bed, he looked at us and declared, 'Jeez, it's like waking to a scene in *The Sopranos*!'

Later on in the day, when Elma and Brian were with him, Donal indicated that he could see Sheila and Mossie, his deceased grandparents, in the room. Throughout his illness, he'd continued to visit their grave and pray for their help and guidance when the time came to leave us.

In the midst of this turmoil, we still had to address practical issues. The chairlift was bulky and awkward when people used the stairs. I contacted the man who had installed it and told him it was time for its removal. True to his word, even though it was Saturday, he came within an hour and the removal was done efficiently, quietly. My heart was hollow as I watched him dismantle it. Donal would not use it again. An hour later, the chairlift and its tracks were gone.

The day wore on. Our house continued to fill with people. Tears flowed and there was laughter also, as we talked about Donal and his short, crammed life. We were advised to rest, but there would be plenty of time for that in the weeks to come. Saturday evening and night were another pain-filled struggle for Donal. We could not make him comfortable. No matter how hard we tried to settle him, he kept slipping down in the bed. We would carefully lift him up, terrified of adding to his discomfort. His bones had become incredibly fragile and could break with any sudden movement. To avoid this, we slid a double sheet under him so that we could ease him into a more comfortable position. On one of these lifts, at around 10 p.m., I heard a crack and knew something had broken. Donal's eyes shot open. They were filled with absolute agony and I prayed for his suffering to end. And yet ... how could we let him go? These conflicting emotions filled our hearts as we counted down these final hours with him.

I remembered a father I'd met in the Ronald McDonald House in the early stages of Donal's illness. His son was on life support and he'd said to me, 'We have to decide whether the plug will be pulled this evening or tomorrow!' What a harrowing decision to have to make, I'd thought at the time. Now I understood the despair that would lead a parent to make such a heart-rending decision.

At an earlier stage, I'd had a discussion with Patricia about the morality around this issue. When the pain became too strong for the drugs to have any effect, and a patient was no longer able to cope with the slightest movement, when should the treatment stop? Was there a justifiable moral reason to continue maintaining life, or should the patient be allowed slip peacefully away without further suffering? Patricia had advised me at the time not to add to my stress by such considerations. 'Don't go there,' she said. But I would have considered going anywhere to stop the pain that was racking my son.

Elma prayed at his bedside, as she had done every evening. While these prayers were being said, a number of texts came through from some friends. *Was Donal okay?* A rumour had started in the town that he had died. I assured the senders that although he was sinking, he was still with us. The night passed in the same limbo-like atmosphere as the previous one. Again, we were advised to go to bed. Donal had an army of loved ones to watch over him, and we would be called if the slightest change in his condition occurred. I managed a little rest and Donal was able to sleep through the night with little movement, except when he was re-aligned in the bed to make him more comfortable.

Sunday morning was a repeat of Saturday. More visitors, even more food, and everyone volunteering to assist where possible. Then, in the late afternoon, people began to drift away. There were cows to be milked, cattle to be fed, jobs to be done at home. Families had to prepare their children for school the following day. Life continued, regardless. It was a strange and quiet parting, as if, deep down, people realised we needed this family time with Donal. By 3.30 p.m., everyone had gone and we were alone.

We sank into the silence that descended over the house. We'd needed the support of friends and family, but it was a relief not to have to talk to anyone, not to have to smile and answer questions. Elma asked if I would sit with Donal for a couple of hours while she rested. She had not slept the previous night and was on the verge of exhaustion. I lay down beside him and chatted to him. I held his hand and promised that his bicycle would be used for the CROSS Rugby Legends Cycle in September, the same cycle he had done the previous year. I thought of the 'bed push' from Dublin to Limerick that we'd planned in such detail. His illness had intervened and it had never taken place. That, too, would be done in his memory. He slept while I talked, occasionally giving my hand a gentle squeeze in response to something I said. I prayed with him and then fell silent. No words were necessary. We were in a place of farewell, but we were not there yet. He was dictating his life right to the end. There would be intense grief when he left us, but no guilt. We had looked into all possible answers, all possible cures, all possible miracles. We had questioned our God as to why our son had to live this life and Donal had answered us when he said, 'Why not!'

At 6.30 p.m., Elma took over and suggested that I try to rest. I was not in the mood for resting. I went downstairs and joined Jema in the conservatory. We settled down together on the sofa and huddled up silently to each other. For almost five years her life had been dominated by Donal's illness and now it was all coming to an end. I knew she would endure those years over and over again, if only she could keep him with her. I cuddled her against me and we watched television together as Elma spent those precious moments with Donal.

Elma is a minister of the Eucharist and at Christmas she and Donal had agreed that she would attend Mass each morning and bring home the Eucharist for him to receive. The Eucharist from Saturday's Mass was still in the house, as Donal had been too weak to swallow it. She knew that this sacred presence was a great consolation to him and told him she would receive it for him. When this was done, she prayed quietly by his side.

At 7 p.m. I went out to call Orla, our family dog. She was lying on the green area across the road from our house. She lifted her head when she heard my voice and began to cross the road. Halfway across, she stiffened and stopped, then turned away from the house. I called her again but she ignored me. She continued to walk up the road in the opposite direction. This was unusual behaviour for an obedient pet dog, house-trained and affectionate. She loved her corner of the conservatory and usually bounded across the road to settle down on her pillow but, now, she just kept going. When she disappeared from view, I took out the jeep and followed her, afraid she would stray too far. When I picked her up, she struggled in my arms and tried to escape. She was obviously distressed and reluctant to get into the jeep. I managed to settle her down and turned the jeep back towards the house. She whimpered as I took her from the jeep and struggled again, becoming even more agitated when I opened the back door and brought her inside. Just as we crossed the threshold, I heard Elma calling for me and for Jema to come quickly to Donal's room. Suddenly, I understood the reason for our dog's uncharacteristic actions. My skin was cold with foreboding as I ran with Jema up the stairs. We'd been expecting this day and looking towards it with dread – yet now that it was happening, we could not believe it.

Donal's breathing had become shallow. Each breath was a struggle. I told Elma to phone Brian, his surrogate father, who was always ready to step in and help when I was working away from home or during those stressful times when Elma and I were in Crumlin, tending to our son. She had already done so and Brian was on his way. We heard the door open downstairs, and his footsteps rushing up towards us. Just as he entered the room, our son took two last gasps and passed peacefully from this world. It was over, as quietly and simply as that. A sigh, and Donal was gone, all suffering ended, his battle done. It was 8 p.m. on a Sunday evening, 12 May 2013. The Feast of the Ascension.

Chapter Fifty
James, John, Cormac and Hugh

'God will be there with His arms open and I'll walk into them.' That's what Donal told us shortly before he died. The last day we saw him, he'd said, 'See you tomorrow, lads,' the way he always did, so we hadn't said goodbye. That's the way he wanted it.

The day he passed away is so vivid still. A few of us had got together and we texted Aislinn. We thought she'd be at home but she was in town with her friend, and they came in her car and collected us. The weather had been mixed all day, with a few showers and wind. We called to James O'Callaghan, who was another friend of Donal's, and we were just hanging around together in his garden, talking about things and wondering if Donal was sleeping. We kept thinking, 'He's hanging in there. He's not going to go, not yet,' – although Elma had tried to prepare us and Fionnbar was keeping in touch with us by phone. Then the clouds opened and the sun slanted down. We went out to the garden and sat there in the brightness. We were talking and having a bit of a laugh together. We figured Donal was sleeping and we were sure he was holding on.

John went around the front of the house to take a call on his mobile. When he came back, he said, 'Lads, that was Fionnbar. Donal's gone.' And those words, 'Donal's gone', they just shocked us into complete silence. It was unbelievable. We really thought he'd beat it again. It was the biggest shock in the world, even though Donal had told us to be ready. We all ran into the hedges and started crying. People say, you must have been prepared for the news but when you're so close to someone, you really can't believe it will actually happen. Then we formed a circle and talked and talked about Donal. Our mums were ringing us, and they came and took us home. The drive home was the worst ever.

It was such a coincidence – the odds of all of us being together at that time, his best friends, girls and lads ... And the sun coming out, like it was a sign Donal was giving us that he was still around. And he is. We have a sense of him about us. If we're sitting exams or playing rugby or football, we feel he's there, pushing us on to do our best. We've met lots of celebrities. They were at Donal's funeral but no matter how inspirational they are, they don't awe us anymore because we've known someone who inspired us more than any of them ever will.

We've special memories of Donal, lots of them. But the saddest thing is that we have more memories to come – but Donal won't be part of them.

Chapter Fifty-One

The death has occurred of Donal WALSH, Hare St, Blennerville, Tralee, Kerry.

WALSH, Donal (Hare Street, Blennerville, Tralee): On 12 May 2013, peacefully, at home, with his devoted parents Fionnbar and Elma, his adored sister Jema and much loved uncle Brian. Sadly missed by his loving family, Granny Mary, aunts, uncles, cousins, relatives and many wonderful friends.

Rest in Peace

House private on Monday. Reposing at Home on Tuesday from 2 p.m. to 8 p.m. Requiem Mass on Wednesday at 12 noon in St John's Church. Burial afterwards in Rath Cemetery. Donations in lieu of flowers to the Palliative Care Unit, Kerry General Hospital and Kare4Kids, care of the Gleasure Funeral Home.

It's strange how the practicalities take over. The phone calls began. We notified Patricia Sheahan, who came over immediately. I could see she was upset as she officially declared that Donal had gone from us. He had passed. I found that term more acceptable. He had simply passed on to another sphere. One where he was free from pain, strong of limb and fleet of foot. It was a comforting thought, as we lingered in his peaceful presence. Those final moments of his life had cured me of any lingering fear of death. Elma felt the same way. The suffering, yes, that was fearsome, but the passing into the light no longer held any terror for us.

Weeks previously, I'd discussed with Graham Gleasure, our local undertaker, what needed to be done when this dreaded moment arrived. It had been a surreal yet pragmatic conversation, akin to a dress rehearsal that we desperately hoped would never make the opening night. Yet that night had arrived and Graham had been expecting my call. Donal had not wanted to leave the house until his coffin was carried out on the funeral walk, and we were anxious to follow his wishes. But we knew he would also want to look his best, as he always did, when showing his face to the public. Those who came to pay their respects – and we knew there would be many – would see only the image of a sporty, normal teenager who had been full of life and vigour. And we, too, wanted to see that Donal. To brand that final memory forever in our hearts. We gathered up the clothes he would wear and entrusted his body for embalming to his final minders, who arrived swiftly at our door. Graham did as we requested and Donal was back with us that night.

We laid our son out in the sitting room. He looked as if he was sleeping. There was a little more gel in his hair than he would have liked but, otherwise, this was the Donal we knew. There was no sign of the pain he had endured for so long and, perhaps, this made us cry all the harder. Our family had gathered in the house to pay their respects. The quiet hush in the sitting room, where people silently prayed, contrasted sharply with the voices from the kitchen as people gathered around the table to talk and offer comfort. Togetherness and endless cups of tea – we do death well in Ireland, and Donal's would be no different.

We quickly realised that word had spread far beyond our family and friends. This is an age of instant communication. Tweets and retweets, Facebook, texts, emails: they all played a part in relaying news of Donal's passing, and word spread like wildfire. Once again Donal Walsh was trending, only this time with the letters 'RIP' after his name. An ironic twist to the trending on Twitter was that Donal had 18,000 followers before he died. On the night of his death that number increased to *24,000*. Did his 6,000 new followers expect a reply? He would have appreciated the irony. I could imagine him flinging back his head and laughing. Yet they were a tribute to him, an indication that his spirit was going to live on in this world of virtual reality.

Another indication that his message was already having an impact, and increasing the level of awareness within sporting bodies, was evidenced by a tweet from Fermoy RFC that read:

Deepest sympathy to the family of Donal Walsh, RIP. Remember, if you need to talk, you have your coaches, manager & friends always available.

But we were too gripped by sorrow to realise exactly what Donal had created through his brief flurry of publicity. All that would become obvious later, and in ways that we could never have anticipated. But for now, we had a wake and a funeral to organise.

The first call on Monday morning was from the office of the President, offering condolences. Later in the morning, Des Healy, Donal's English teacher, arrived and told us that a wall in the school with his writings, and all the articles written about him, had been set up as a tribute to him. The oratory had been dedicated to him for the next few days, so that the students could write notes of condolences and memories of times they had spent with him.

I returned to the school with Des to acknowledge the tributes. I needed a break from the overwhelming grief I felt every time I entered the sitting room and looked at Donal, as I had done so often in the past when he was just stirring from sleep. That same sadness hung over the school. I examined the wall of tributes and entered the oratory. A picture of Donal had been placed in the centre of the room. Boys entered and stood for a few minutes in meditation, before slipping the notes they had written into a bowl and leaving just as quietly. It was eerie, this silence hanging over the corridors that normally rang with the energy of 600 boys. Des asked if I would meet with some of Donal's pals, who were very upset. I sat with them and recounted his final hours, reassured them that he had embraced death bravely and with dignity.

Three of the boys who had been in his rugby squad were particularly distressed. As they had been so close to Donal, I invited them to the house after school for a private visit. One of these was Danny Cournane, a young boy with an Irish/Maori background. Danny always performed the Haka prior to every game the team played in their West Munster League. Donal had been his rugby mentor and Danny had played his heart out on the pitch for him. He arranged to visit with his mother that afternoon. When they arrived and were paying their respects, I had a sudden thought. Donal had loved watching Danny do the Haka. What if it could be performed at his funeral? Danny smiled at the notion and said it was something he'd love to do as a tribute. Elma was passing the room at the time and when I mentioned this possibility to her, she agreed that it should form part of the funeral rituals.

Later that morning, my brother Andrew rang and asked if the pallbearers of Donal's coffin had been chosen. All such arrangements had already been made and I'd worked closely with my friend Jay Galvin, who, with two other friends, was organising the practical details. We were anxious that all those close to Donal would have a role to play in the service. But, according to Andrew, things were already changing. Paul O'Connell had been in touch to offer his condolences but now a request had come from Donal's beloved Munster team – those who were free wanted to attend the funeral and participate at some level in the ceremony. This was an honour we'd never expected and we were deeply moved by the request. I reckoned Donal, if he was watching from on high, was grinning from ear to ear at this unexpected acknowledgement from his heroes.

And so the day continued. Several hundred people from the locality passed through our house. Tomorrow would be a public day, and we were already aware that this was going to bring an even larger number of visitors. As so many young people were calling, we made a decision that no alcohol was to be served. But the food kept coming. Our friend, Maura O'Sullivan, had gathered together a small army who catered to everyone's needs and a number of businesses in Tralee sent complimentary trays of food.

When Fr Francis Nolan arrived that night to organise the funeral service for Wednesday, Elma said she would like to give the eulogy. I would be carrying Donal's coffin and laying him to rest. For me, the physical task was easier. I probably could not have stood in front of a crowded church without breaking down. But I knew that Elma, who had been so staunch throughout Donal's illness, would find the strength to honour our son in this way.

The following morning we were awoken by a phone call from the office of the Taoiseach. Enda Kenny offered his condolences to Elma, who accepted them with gratitude and held a brief conversation with him. Thus began a day that brought about 2,000 people to our house to pay their respects to Donal. They came from sports organisations – including footballers and rugby players whom Donal had worshipped – there were my work colleagues and people from Elma's company, there were strangers who had heard his message and been moved by his courage.

I don't know how our friends catered for everyone. Thoughts of the loaves and fishes came to my mind as I looked out the window, where a small marquee had been set up in the front garden. The wind blows hard from the mountains in this part of the world and the marquee offered protection against the weather to those who were patiently waiting outside.

'Mom, will people remember me?' Donal had asked Elma, shortly after his cancer had been declared terminal.

I guess he knew the answer by now.

Later that night, when the visitors had left and the house was quiet again, Fr Raymond Browne, the yet-to-be-ordained but newly appointed Bishop of Kerry, arrived with two priests from the diocese. They spoke to us about Donal's contribution to the much-needed discussion on suicide and its impact. But we also had some light-hearted banter as Elma, who is a parochial minister, chatted with the local priests about late nights in 'the Abbey'. Did our newly appointed Bishop realise they were talking about the Christmas parties in Tralee's famous late night bar and not Tralee's equally famous Holy Cross Priory? Another day had ended and the final night's vigil with Donal began.

Chapter Fifty-Two

He wore a suit and a red tie. Fashion conscious to the end. And his friends, when they arrived, were dressed identically. Little keepsakes were placed beside him in his coffin: his favourite aftershave and deodorant, his Zippo (a friend had given this elegant lighter to him at Christmas, so that he could whip it out and offer to light a girl's cigarette). Jema requested to keep Huskie, a fluffy toy dog that Donal had never abandoned as he grew older, and which we had laid beside him for last two days. The lads and Aislinn said their goodbyes, and then it was his cousins' turn to bid him a tearful farewell. Finally, just Elma, Jema, my uncle Bill, my mother, Mary, and Donal's uncles were left alone with him. Prayers were said by his uncle, Fr Michael, as each of us said our last goodbyes. The silence surrounding Donal deepened into an impenetrable sadness as his coffin was closed.

Nothing prepares you for the reality of that moment, the sheer physical separation. That tearing apart is as painful as the rending of a heart. But we had a funeral to attend and so we gathered ourselves together and carried his coffin to the waiting hearse. We gathered behind it and held on to each other as we began the long walk behind his coffin to the church.

The morning was sunny and only a few clouds shadowed the peaks of Slieve Mish. The canal sparkled as it reflected the sun back at us. We made up a small crowd of about fifty mourners as we left the house. All of us, as a sign of unity, wore a red ribbon. Across the road, television cameras followed our progress. They did not intrude and we were hardly aware of their presence. An Garda Síochána had blocked all traffic from the bridge and two squad cars were waiting to lead the cortege into Tralee. As we rounded the bend, we saw the first guard of honour. Donal's rugby and 'Naries' teammates, and pupils from his school were lined up in two files on either side of the road. In all, about a hundred or so young people were waiting to accompany him to his final resting place.

The procession paused for a few moments outside the Kerins O'Rahillys club, where more young 'Naries' had gathered. They silently joined the procession. As the hearse began to move on, we heard a round of applause from onlookers. This gesture was repeated wherever people had gathered to pay their respects. We passed the Bon Secours Hospital where the earlier stages of his illness had been played out. Most of the medical staff had come out to applaud his courage. At the Brogue Inn we received a similar salute from the crowds lining the street. It was only then that we realised all the businesses had closed down for the duration of Donal's funeral – the local shops, the international high-fashion outlets, the banks, the cafes and bistros, and the offices – all had closed their doors and the staff were waiting outside to bid farewell to Donal.

As we moved up the Mall, which, with its hotels and business premises, is normally a hive of activity and a ceaseless flow of cars, we were greeted by a street devoid of traffic. The only sound I could hear was the squeak of a sign above a doorway. And then a ripple of applause as the crowd swelled on either side of the street. When we arrived at the gates of St John's Church, we realised there was no way everyone would fit inside. It was later estimated that between 5,000 and 7,000 people had arrived to attend Donal's farewell Mass and no one was leaving until the end.

His friends, John, James, Cormac and Hugh, with his cousins Eoin and Ríos, carried his coffin from the gates to the doors of the church. How strong they looked, how healthy. The ache in our hearts was indescribable as we watched these young men shoulder him high. At the entrance to the church my brothers Michael, Thomás, Seán, Andrew, Kieran and I took over and brought him to the altar. Everyone stood to attention as we passed by. In the midst of the crowd, I saw his beloved Munster squad dressed in their formal blazers and ties and thought, 'There you go, Donal. They're with you to the very end.'

The ceremony was simple and began with a letter of condolence that had been handed to me by Colonel Brendan McAndrew, President Higgins' aide-de-camp. Then Donal's friends carried symbols of his life to the altar. Shane Jennings presented a rugby jersey, in recognition of his love of sport. Paul Galvin presented a pen and paper, as a symbol of his writing, and John Kelly carried his Local Hero Award. These were placed near his coffin and the Mass commenced. The singing by Donal's school choir and his friend, Andrew Grey, was magnificent. Fr Francis spoke about Donal's witness to his faith, his value on life and his dignity in his final illness. He urged young people to remember Donal's message, to think twice before committing an act that would have such far-reaching and tragic consequences.

At the end of the service Elma delivered the eulogy. Two weeks before Donal died, she had written it in an hour, the words flowing from her. At the last minute she had added a section, on the forthcoming G8 summit which was due to take place the following month in Fermanagh. She called on the government to use their influence at the summit to commit more funding to cancer research. The previous day when the Taoiseach, Enda Kenny rang, she had spoken to him about the statistics of cancer recovery, which now has a 60 to 70 per cent cure rate. Our son had lost the odds on those statistics, and a cure had to be found to prevent other families suffering the loss of a loved one, as we had done.

When Mass ended, the officers of Tralee RFC stood by the coffin as a guard of honour, while the remaining mourners came to sympathise with us. This ritual of condolence was so long that my nephew had to use the bathroom. When he returned, he discovered he was standing between members of the Munster rugby team.

'See, I told you that one day you'd line out with Munster,' his father whispered in his ear. Donal would have roared laughing at the joke, especially as the lad in question was a Leinster mini-rugby player! What is it about Irish funerals that one can laugh and cry in the same breath? John, my friend who had flown from Scotland to be with us, joked that he'd seen the queue outside the church and thought he might be missing something. But once inside, he couldn't get out.

An estimated 3,000 people had shaken our hands by the time the queue dwindled and we were free to leave the church. I had to sympathise with the Tralee RFC guard of honour, who stood stoically to attention throughout the hour-and-a-half while we were receiving these condolences.

Elma's brothers, Maurice, Donal, Johnny, Brian, Brendan and I carried Donal away from the altar to the doors of the church where his Munster heroes bore him to the hearse. This was something special and while Donal would have been embarrassed by all that was happening, he would also have been absolutely chuffed – especially when Danny Cournane stepped out of the crowd and did his Irish version of the traditional Haka.

Danny had studied the ritual Maori grieving tradition and given it an Irish twist. In the true tradition of this ceremonial rite, the person chosen to perform the Haka sits for twenty-four hours with the body of his dead comrade or loved one and fasts during that time. He then offers a gift of food to the mourners. Obviously, we did not expect Danny to fast. Instead he came to present us with his gift – his own jersey signed by all his team, the team Donal had trained. I'd managed to hold myself together until that moment but I almost broke when he reached into the jersey he was wearing and pulled out his West Munster League medal of that year and declared, 'I would not have this medal but for Donal. Now I wish to return it to you. It is my gift in appreciation for the life of your son.' Then he stood in front of the hearse and did an outstanding Haka. The poise of this fourteen-year-old boy was astonishing, and the incredible energy of his performance will long be remembered in Tralee and far beyond.

On the way to the graveyard, cars and buses stopped, the passengers alighted and applauded as we passed. At the railway station the photographers slipped away and we were left on our own, removed at last from the media glare. This was a mixed blessing, as I had one final duty to perform. It would have had a wider impact if it had been caught on film, but I wanted the publicity for only one reason: to hammer home Donal's message to the widest possible group of his peers.

We placed his coffin on the wooden slats that spanned the grave and Fr Michael, my brother, officiated at the graveside. He recited the final prayers and Donal was slowly lowered into the earth. Graham, the undertaker, was about to place the grass matting over the grave, as is the usual custom. Not this time.

'Where are the shovels?' I asked Graham. 'We have ten uncles and five friends, along with myself. Together, we will bury my son.'

I wanted those young people standing around the graveside to understand the full significance of Donal's message. He had called suicide 'a permanent solution to a temporary problem', and these teenagers would see that there was *no* coming back from death. No fake glass would hide this raw truth. Death by suicide is not a topic to be glorified on Facebook and Twitter. This was a grave, a deep hole with no way out. And so we buried my son, with shovels, sweat and tears.

Chapter Fifty-Three
Extract from Elma's Eulogy

Abraham Lincoln once said, 'It is the not the years in your life that count, it is the life in your years' – and that is so true of Donal. From the day he was born, he could not wait to catch up to his big sister, Jema. He had to be better at spelling, reading, running, football, and on and on ... He once asked her not to learn to drive before him ... and she didn't! She was always so patient and kind to him, more especially in the past few months. Donal would ask her to open this, get that, do the other and, patiently, she would do it for him. Jema is the best big sister anyone could ask for and when she got Donal for a brother, God knew what He was doing ...

In the nearly seventeen years we have known Donal, I don't think he ever sat down for long. He was always on the go – even if it was a trip to the cinema, he would be in and out about four times. He loved organising outings with the lads; trips to the shops and of course the big trips to London and Paris, where he had the time of his life with everyone; trips to concerts, and of course birthday parties. Anything that was on, he was there.

I don't think there is a person here who did not benefit from Donal's generosity in some form. His recent interview on RTÉ and the write-up he did in the *Sunday Independent* touched the hearts of the nation and the letters we have received are a testament to this. The gifts he bought for his family and friends – he was always a generous boy. One time when he was about nine years old, we were in a shop when I bumped into a cousin and her two kids. Donal had a bar of chocolate in his hand and was about to eat it. I looked around and he was gone – back he came with another two bars for her children, unknown to me. 'Now I can eat my chocolate,' he said.

Those of us who really knew Donal knew he wasn't ever shy in what he wanted. When he didn't get his way, like any normal teenager, we got the normal pouting and slamming of doors. But more than all the gifts he gave, it was his nature and smile that most people will remember him for. He always had kind words for everyone, even in the depths of his pain and suffering. He had great time for his family and friends. His loyalty to all his friends and family was very important to him.

While today Donal is known for his stance on suicide, it is important to remember Donal died from one of the biggest modern-day killers. Cancer. While suffering this disease, Donal was an ambassador for cancer awareness and advocated at national and international level, even to the United Nations, to increase research and funding into this killer disease. If he was alive today, he would be the first to support me in asking the upcoming G8 summit to increase funding and advance possible cures for cancer.

Donal also had a great sense of spirituality and faith: this meant a lot to him and he wanted the best for everyone he met. Donal once said to me that he didn't mind dying early, once he went to heaven with a clean spirit. We can safely say he never had an enemy and cared for all those who got to know him. To the young people here, we say, 'Live every day to the full and carry on his spirit in your lives, just as his lightning spirit struck you in his brief time with us ...'

Fionnbar, Jema, Brian and myself will miss Donal all the days of our life and now wish for him a peaceful rest in the arms of God, till we meet again.

We love you, Donal.

PART TWO
REMEMBERING DONAL

Chapter Fifty-Four
2013–2014

The aftermath is shattering. I never imagined otherwise. Exhaustion struggles with grief, as I try to settle down following the exacting days of Donal's wake and funeral. Everywhere I look, I see reminders of him. Even the view from our kitchen window is dominated by the mountains that symbolised his final journey. There's so much to be done. The thought of dealing with any of it is tough, but we have to keep busy. Elma looks after the official paperwork, while I return the equipment that was installed for his final illness. His bed is made. It seems to be waiting for him to pull back the duvet and settle down for a good night's sleep. But even though the sterile atmosphere of sickness has vanished, along with the syringes, medicines and oxygen, the room remains an empty space that nothing seems capable of filling. Have we moved too quickly to banish all signs of his illness? Have we allowed ourselves time to absorb and process those harrowing months? Probably not. We're striving to return some normality to our lives, but is that possible when a young person in a family dies? I doubt it.

Each stage of his short life will be engraved in my memory until I die. Our sturdy, active baby, his blond fringe falling over his blue eyes. Even then, those eyes had a compelling curiosity. The young boy, growing taller than his peers, his head bent so that he could join in their conversations. My pride as I watched from the sidelines as he led from the front and passed the ball so that others could make the score. And then the unthinkable, the slow realisation that pitiless things happen. Now, all we can do is create a new routine, a different order. That will be an individual experience for each of us. Like our grief. We support each other in turn. One is strong while the other falters and vice versa. But we each endure our cross in our own private way. We're devastated, yet the sun still rises and sets, the world keeps turning. And outside forces are already at play.

On the day after the funeral, Billy Keane, a local journalist with the *Irish Independent*, calls to our house. Donal's funeral moved him deeply and he'd like to write a feature about our son and the den where Donal spent so much of his time. I've met Billy before. His son and Donal played football against each other. I lead him towards Donal's Make-A-Wish den and leave him there. I'm not ready to look at the numerous scrawled signatures, the quirky, sometimes profound sayings that his friends scribbled on the walls. Or to read the words Donal stencilled high above us: 'Each day is a gift. It's not a given right.' His drums are silent and that is more than I can bear.

I've always enjoyed reading Billy's features, especially his reports on the Munster games, and I know he'll write a strong feature on Donal. On the following Saturday, it's published on the front page of the *Irish Independent*, with a picture of Donal. His wide smile and steady gaze – he was never camera shy. Billy phones to tell me about the positive reaction the feature received.

'All down to Donal,' he says, and I remember the words Brendan O'Connor used on *The Saturday Night Show* at the end of his interview: 'You know what, Donal, when you do go, I know you're going to leave a great legacy behind.'

At the time those words went over my head in the general excitement of the night and the distressing weeks that followed. But I hear them now and they grow louder with each letter that arrives to our address. These letters have grown in number since his passing. More than half of them contain donations, and requests that we pass the money on to Donal's charities. Teenagers, mainly transition-year students, ask our permission to fundraise in his memory. They are encouraging their schools to organise mental health awareness weeks. Strangers travel across the country to visit Donal's grave. Each time we visit the cemetery, we find more new cards, notes or flowers placed there by people who never knew him but feel a connection to his spirit. One man travels from Tipperary and knocks on our door. 'Just to give Donal's mom a hug,' he says, and leaves when this is done.

Brendan is right. Donal has left a legacy behind. It needs to be preserved but I don't know how this will be done or what the future holds for us, when we're in the grip of such terrible grief. Yet, somehow, I know that our son's story has not come to an end. In Gleasure's Funeral Home, I hear about a woman who drove from Cork on the day of his funeral to hand in a donation for the charities we'd chosen in lieu of flowers. Then, not wishing to intrude on the funeral, she turned around and drove home. She and many others like her have contributed over €3,000 in funeral fund donations for the Palliative Care Unit in Kerry General and Kare4Kids. Graham will leave the account open for another few weeks. In the end the funeral contributions total over €5,000.

It's strange how stories such as these lift my spirits, even briefly. I can even laugh when I hear about the call Graham received from RTÉ on the day of Donal's funeral. It was unrelated to Donal, and the person who rang from the television station was in need of some urgent information and wanted to deal only with Graham. The first call came at 10 a.m. and the calls continued every two hours throughout the day. Each time Graham had still not returned to his office. Finally, in frustration, the caller asked, 'What kind of funerals do you have in Kerry, that go on all day long?' To which the answer was, 'Donal's funeral.'

As it happened, Graham did not return to his office until after 5 p.m. that evening. By his reckoning it was the longest he had ever worked on any one funeral. As Jay Galvin remarked when we finally laid Donal to rest, 'That's as close as Tralee is going to see to a state funeral for a long time to come.'

Elma and I return to work. It's important to have a structure to our days and we're treated with great kindness by our respective employers. We're doing as Donal requested – trying to move on to the next stage of our lives. Work is therapeutic and gives us a reason for rising in the mornings. But as each day passes, the full enormity of what we've lost weighs more heavily on us. Donal's passing has allowed us to finally release our pent-up emotions. We no longer have to pretend to be brave and resolute and optimistic. We can cry and not try to hide our tears, for fear they will upset the positivity Donal built around himself. So we cry an ocean on the bad days and on the days when we are calm, we talk about his legacy and what we must do to nurture it.

Towards the end of May, Donal is nominated for a posthumous Rehab People of the Year Award. His name has been put forward by Radio Kerry and the South Kerry Coroner, Terence Casey. The results will be announced in September 2013. To get to September without falling apart seems an impossibility, yet one day follows another and things keep happening.

The Kerry Group re-name their Annual Crumlin Golf Classic in Donal's name. Henceforth it will be called the Donal Walsh Crumlin Golf Classic. In the lush green surrounds of the Killarney Golf and Fishing Club, Elma and I pose for photographs. The day is beautiful, a clear blue sky and soaring temperatures. Nothing *Angela's Ashes* about the summer of 2013. Ronan O'Gara officially launches the tournament. The last time we saw him, he was shouldering our son's coffin. We're pleased to see him, grateful to him for the heartening attention he gave to Donal during his struggle. The tournament will raise €30,000 in Donal's name for Crumlin Hospital. There is definitely something stirring in the air.

In June, we celebrate his seventeenth birthday with his Month's Mind Mass. The church is crowded with hundreds of people who have come to pray with us and mark the first month of Donal's passing. Afterwards, we fly to Oporto in Portugal for a week. This will be our first holiday without him. I'm anxious as we pack, unsure how we will manage, especially Jema. They were never easy on each other, one giving as good as the other when it came to banter and teasing, but they were best friends, confidants and holiday companions. I wish I could take Jema's grief and banish it. And do the same with Elma's tears, which she sheds every day. I wish I could wake up and discover this was all a dream.

An unexpected invitation arrives before we leave. We became used to people's generosity when Donal was alive – the helicopter rides and overnight stays in luxurious hotels. We don't expect that to continue, yet here is an invitation to stay in the K Club golf resort in Kildare on our way out. We accept the invitation and, in the lavish presidential suite, we enjoy the moment and wallow in luxury. I so appreciate this kindly gesture, especially for Jema's sake. She never resented the 'spoiling' Donal received, but now she has an opportunity to enjoy a little bit of 'spoiling' herself.

In Portugal we relax and allow ourselves to be tired. For the first few days, all we are capable of doing is lounging around and sleeping late. At night we eat by the cobbled harbour and watch the slow roll of the Douro river, where boats list under barrels of port and the old, red-roofed houses rise in glittering tiers above us. This is a restful place, where we can gather our strength for the future. I hire a mountain bike and begin my training programme. The promise I made to Donal in those final, precious hours we spent together has not been forgotten. I will take part in the CROSS Rugby Legends Cycle in September.

This is my first time to cycle seriously in twenty-five years. It's tough going, especially on the hills, but I grit my teeth and keep pedalling. I manage about 30 kilometres every morning and am already feeling fitter by the time we return home. I'm determined to participate in the cycle, as Donal did the previous year, and raise funds for cancer research. A 60 to 70 per cent cure rate is simply not good enough.

We take a trip to Compostela, the destination of the famous Camino de Santiago pilgrimage. I've wanted to see the Cathedral of Santiago de Compostela for a long time. We drive the 300 kilometres to our destination but the weather is cold and, somehow, we are not in the mood for exploring. After a visit to the cathedral, the reputed burial place of Saint James, we return to Oporto and take it easy before undertaking our next long drive.

Ten years previously, when we visited the shrine of Fatima, Donal was with us. Six years old and curious, he was enthralled by the story of the three shepherd children who saw the apparitions of Mary and refused to be swayed from their belief, despite bullying and threats. This is a bittersweet return journey for all of us. Here, nothing has changed. The statues of the three children still dominate the entrance to the shrine, the basilica remains a silent place of pilgrimage while, outside, small shops and stalls overflow with wax candles and effigies. I was deeply moved by the experience when I first came here, and I still feel the same surge of emotion as we stand on the spot where the apparitions took place. My faith is strong and never wavered during those tumultuous years of Donal's illness, when it seemed as if God was looking the other way.

We head out of town to visit Aljustrel, where the houses of the three children are located. Two died young: Francisco and Jacinta. I think of them as we stand outside their houses. Influenza – that was the killer disease in those days.

Elma's name is called as we are about to enter the first house. A close friend who was unable to attend Donal's funeral has arrived with her family, two young people about the same age as Jema. Her husband died some years previously, also from cancer, and we have much to talk about. We spend the afternoon together, astounded at the coincidence of meeting in such unfamiliar surroundings. We originally planned on visiting Fatima on Thursday and they intended doing the trip on Friday. Yet we are both here on Wednesday at exactly the same time. Is Donal pulling strings? Little things keep happening. Symbolic or coincidental, it hardly seems to matter.

Another day on the beach when Jema is playing his iTunes collection, a song he loved comes on – just as a turquoise jumper, identical to his favourite one, floats in on the tide. We watch it sway on the crest of a wave then drift away again. He is with us in spirit if not in person, we believe, and that thought consoles us. But music is the undoing of me, especially when I hear the songs he loved, like Phil Coulter's 'Home from the Sea'. His strong voice rising, as we drove home from Thomond Park.

Home, home, home from the sea,
Angels of mercy, answer our plea.
And carry us home, home, home from the sea
Carry us safely home, from the sea.

When we return home, Elma and I are interviewed on radio by Miriam O'Callaghan. It is a raw, powerful interview and we find it difficult to speak without breaking down. Miriam is a sensitive interviewer and what is supposed to last approximately twenty minutes goes on for almost an hour. This results in another deluge of calls, letters, more donations. The momentum grows. A TV3 televised interview follows. Brendan invites us back on *The Saturday Night Show* to talk about Donal and how we are coping in the aftermath of his passing. Donal's story refuses to go away and he has left us with the challenge of nurturing his legacy.

Donations sometimes come from wealthy contributors but they are also offered by people living on the borderline of poverty. One woman existing solely on her old age pension sends us €70. A property developer who wants to remain anonymous sends us €5,000. Each donation is equally appreciated, but how do we take on the responsibility of ensuring that this money is channelled in the right direction? We're trying to cope with our terrible grief, yet if people are willing to take their hard-earned euros from their limited budgets and send them on to us, we have to respond, somehow. Donal has thrown a stone into a pond and the ripples have become a tidal wave.

Chapter Fifty-Five

One day, while we're still struggling to deal with this tide of generosity, my boss Patrick calls me into his office. He understands that we're going through a time of great sorrow and adjustment, but he believes it's necessary to create a structure that will honour Donal's legacy in a practical, long-lasting way. He's afraid such a suggestion may seem insensitive so soon after Donal's passing, but I realise he's right. We need a plan of action to respond to the goodwill surrounding us. This is how the idea, of establishing a foundation to support the charities Donal always championed, begins.

Patrick believes that the 2013 Summerfest in Killarney would be the ideal event to launch the foundation. Elma and I discuss this possibility. An opportunity we never sought has been presented to us. It seems like an answer to our prayers, but is it a road we want to take? Will we be able for the continuing publicity that, even now, is eating into so much of our time? Are we strong enough to cope with the organisation and planning that will be necessary to develop a Donal Walsh foundation?

After much discussion, we both agree that it is our way forward and Summerfest will provide the perfect platform to promote it. Donal is helping us to focus on the future. If we can highlight the issue of youth suicide and save lives, then we are acknowledging the importance of his message.

We decide on a name for the foundation and quietly register it. We are blessed with the assistance of a strong marketing team who generously donate their time to help us. We discover, quite by accident, that on the day following Donal's appearance on *The Saturday Night Show*, someone registered the domain 'Donalwalsh.org'. We have no intention of buying that domeain back, so instead we decide on the most common tagline used when his interview with Brendan trended on Twitter – 'Live Life'. We believe those two simple words capture Donal's message, and so www.donalwalshlivelife.org is registered.

Donal's foundation will have two functions. He once told Elma that he would live with the pain of cancer until he was eighty years old, if only he was offered that option. But it was a choice which was not open to him, so his message will now be passed on through other channels: word-of-mouth, the print and broadcast media, social media and visits by Elma and myself to schools and other venues, to talk about Donal and his plea to young people. To pass on his anti-suicide message will not require much funding. The second, equally important, aim of the foundation will be to continue the fundraising that started so spontaneously after his death and donate these funds to appropriate charities. The foundation also hopes to assist families who were trying to deal with a child's life-threatening illness. The costs that can occur when parents are at their most distressed and vulnerable are often unexpected and demanding. We had first-hand experience of these costs and would not have managed, except for the incredible support we received.

From small beginnings, our foundation grows. We establish a board of directors and a committee, who decide on the appropriate charities to support. The Donal Walsh #Livelife Foundation is launched at Summerfest. A gala ball is held, a teddy bears' picnic enjoyed by the little ones and there is a youths' cycle event, open to young people over the age of ten: all are organised in Donal's memory.

Running the foundation takes up an incredible amount of our time. We are on a sharp learning curve, especially when it comes to delegating. Otherwise, we would be swamped by the requests we receive to organise fundraising events in Donal's name. Many volunteer groups manage and run their own events to support the foundation. Some schools are currently organising #Livelife Health weeks. This has been at the instigation of the pupils, who are anxious to spread the message of mental health awareness among young people. We're willing to support all these ventures where possible, and appreciate each and every effort made to support us. But we are very conscious that we must bring some regularity back to our family lives, and find the courage to deal with the emptiness of Donal's physical absence.

We've decided to organise a number of annual fundraising events under the #Livelife banner. These will include Climb Donal's Mountain – a climb up Mount Brandon in west Kerry, which Elma will lead. The CrossDonalsMountain cycle will cover the Kerry stage of the CROSS Cycle, with all proceeds going to the CROSS Foundation. We will hold a #Livelife Celeb Am Golf Classic and a #Livelife Charity Challenge which will involve young people, particularly transition-year students.

Invitations to speak at various functions continue to arrive. Usually, I accept such invitations on Monday, my day off. Elma is free on Thursdays and Fridays, and we are constantly visiting schools and community centres. Elma can speak with confidence about caring for a sick child. She knows what it's like to lie on a roll-out bed beside her son in the same small room, while a thin curtain separates them from a child or a baby struggling to breathe. She has seen a distraught mother, her young daughter clasped in her arms as she carried her to the morgue. This scene, witnessed while she was standing in the corridor outside Donal's ward, is seared into her memory.

I too have witnessed much. I'll never forget the conversation I had with a father whose four-year-old son had been given an 'all clear' prognosis. Six weeks later, we met again. Things had changed drastically in that time and the little boy had relapsed with a very aggressive form of cancer. Two days later, I was praying beside his body in the hospital morgue. He was laid out on a white sheet and looked as if he was resting in his jeans, check shirt and trainers. After the prayers ended, he was laid in his mother's arms as she sat into the back of their family car. His father was going to drive him home. Remembering the tormented drives I'd taken when we received bad news about Donal, I appealed to this man's brothers not to let him drive.

'This is the last thing that he can do for his only child and he is determined to drive him home,' one of them replied. Sometimes, it is wiser to remain silent.

Off they went on their heartbroken journey and I was left with the image of that cheerful little boy, whom I'd met for the first time only a few months earlier in the Ronald McDonald House. Yes, we have profound memories that only those who have undergone a similar loss can truly appreciate. But we mostly talk about Donal and his upbeat attitude to life.

The requests that come our way are not sectarian. We've been contacted by many different religious groups, including the Muslim community. Elma enjoys meeting young people across the country and believes they are responsible, through their fundraising endeavours, for 60 per cent of the donations #Livelife receives. Recently, at the end of one of her talks, she was approached by a young girl in tears. It turned out that she and Donal had become friends when he was in the Gaeltacht. This young student had wonderful, happy photographs to share with Elma, who cherishes all such encounters.

The letters continue to arrive. It seems as if Donal's honesty acted as a catalyst that allows people to bare their souls and open themselves up to us in ways we could never have imagined. Some of the letters make us weep. Elma is particularly moved by one young girl who writes: 'God does not know my address.' What powerful, desperate words. What has she gone through in her life, to bring her to a stage where she feels bereft of any spiritual comfort? We read harrowing stories of loneliness, childhood traumas, and the loss of beloved children who have taken their own lives. Many describe battles with depression and mental illness – and the writers of such letters are glad Donal added his voice to this important debate. His real legacy is to ensure that this conversation continues, and that is what we are doing through the Donal Walsh #Livelife Foundation.

Chapter Fifty-Six

I keep cycling and follow a rigorous training schedule. I'm now able to cycle up to 60 kilometres at a stretch. I remember how Donal used to play the drums. How he would practise obsessively until the tempo was perfect and, also, when he knew his cancer had returned, how he channelled his anguish into that frantic beat, before his shoulder became too sore to play. My feet pedal with that same pent-up energy. The terrain is tough and demanding, particularly the hills. It seems that no matter how many I manage to climb, there is always another one rising in the distance. Is this a metaphor for those final four years of Donal's life? I write to him about my struggles on the bike. Somehow, it seems to help. It's therapeutic and I'm able to laugh as I imagine him reading my complaints, my belly-aching about hills and my tender muscles. He knows what I'm enduring. He did it himself. The only difference is that he did it to fight for his life. I'm doing it to honour that fight. So I keep training in Bantry on my off-duty hours and in Tralee when I'm at home. I return exhausted from the ride but calmer, wiped out, and ready to rest.

July 2013

Hi Donal,

Missed out on my visit to you on my Monday cycle, but I do have an excuse! I had intended as my route to hit Moll's Gap from home, to see how bad that particular run really is. Killarney was no problem and then I headed up towards the gap but a mist closed in and, after the sunshine of the previous weeks, made the road very slippy, and I felt the bike give a few times. 'Might need new tyres soon,' I thought. It was getting bad a couple of kilometres below Ladies View and I then put safety first and decided I wasn't going to trust coming down in this, as it might be too dangerous – so I turned back. At this stage I had gone about nine of the seventeen kilometres from Killarney.

Got back to town safely and the ominous-looking clouds were threatening to break the summer we had enjoyed for the last month, so I took cover until they blew over or it rained. After about thirty minutes it looked safe to move on and so I did. I had just done about one mile when I heard the most distressing sound ever – Psssshhhhh! Yep, you have guessed it: a puncture on the back wheel. That is when I realised how unprepared this 'cyclist' really is. I had no repair kit, no spare tube, no pump and, worst of all, I even forgot my mobile phone! Here I was, stuck a mile at the wrong side of Killarney, and none of the above. I started walking back to town when, nearing the roundabout, who should turn up only Pam Barret, from rugby! An angel in disguise who picked me and the bike up, and carried us home. Think the lesson here is: 'Fulfil your commitment to your son, or get punished by the puncture – but even he relents and sends an angel.'

Talk soon –

Dad

8 August 2013

Hi Donal,

Okay, this bike thing is getting serious. I went out on Tuesday with Chris and a couple of guys from Tralee Chain Gang, and clocked up 64k in 2 hours and 25 minutes. Then on Saturday, myself and John from the hotel took on Caha once more. 54K in one hour and 52 minutes. We are getting fairly good at this but I'm really beginning to appreciate where you had got to in such a short time, with prosthetic knee and only two-thirds lung capacity.

When we were coming down from Caha, we could see the weather begin to change and so we didn't force the brakes too much, in an effort to beat it. Hit Glengarriff and all was well, but the clouds were getting darker, so kept motoring and then, when we just arrived at Ballylickey, the heavens opened. Bad enough the flies, bad enough the wind but this rain bucketed down so much that the glasses were not able to cope. I would have needed wipers on full blast to even see a little of where we were going. It didn't matter – we just were so wet, we trudged on to Bantry and the lads in the hotel had a grand laugh at the two sopping mid-life crises that returned from their ride!

Ah well, another day tomorrow.

Talk soon –

Dad

Chapter Fifty-Seven

It's time for the real thing. The CROSS Rugby Legends Cycle started off as an Irish event, organised by Paul and David Wallace, both retired Irish rugby union legends. Cycling is seen as a vigorous alternative for many who retire from playing rugby. It needs strength but does not make demands on strained joints. What began as an enjoyable exercise among friends soon developed a more serious purpose and the CROSS Rugby Legends Cycle was set up to raise funds for cancer research. It has grown in stature since its inception, and almost everyone involved in this demanding journey from Malin Head to Mizen Head has a story to tell about a loved one lost through this dreadful disease. Some stories are utterly heartbreaking, especially the ones I hear about brave, precious children, whose pattern of cancer followed Donal's story and ended with the same tragic loss.

The CROSS Cycle now attracts international rugby players, and the participants in the September 2013 cycle include legends like Anton Oliver, who earned fifty-nine caps playing for the All Blacks, and David Campese, capped 101 times for Australia. On the home front, renowned legends like Aidan Murphy, Eric Elwood, Shane O'Dwyer and Mick Galwey are among the elite group who undertake the journey. It will start in the most northerly point of Donegal and make its way down the length of Ireland, with cyclists joining in at various stages. I've worked with Michael O'Boyle, the team manager for the cycle, to get the balance of the Kerry stage exactly right. Participants can do half a stage, from Tralee to Moll's Gap, or the full 110-kilometre round trip.

The training has not got any easier but I'm fit enough to do the Sean Kelly 100-kilometre cycle as a test run. I last the distance and cycle it in under four hours. As a result, I should be able to last the pace. I'll ride to Moll's Gap and continue on to Bantry with the riders who are going on to the next stage and staying overnight in the Maritime Hotel. The name of the Kerry stage has been changed to the CrossDonalsMountain. I'm happy with the title. It could not be more perfect.

When the CROSS Cycle Legends reach Tralee, they are met by a welcoming committee that includes myself and Elma, and the overjoyed pupils of CBS The Green. Calling into schools at the different stages and interacting with the pupils is part of the CROSS Cycle journey, and the CBS boys now have a chance to mingle with their heroes.

On the morning after Donal died, I stood here and read the tributes from his fellow students. I was dazed then and had no idea how I would move forward again. At times, I'm still bewildered by all that happened, but there is now a purpose to my life and I must thank him for it. I address the pupils who knew him so well and tell them about the work we are doing in his memory.

Over 150 cyclists of all ages – male and female – join me the following morning to begin the CrossDonalsMountain stage. They include Donal's close friends and many pupils from his school. We set out from the rugby club at 8 a.m. and stop outside our house for a minute's silence. That same silence is observed as we pass the graveyard where Donal's body rests. We know his spirit is with us, urging us onwards. The jerseys we wear were designed and approved by Donal, with the colours pink for breast cancer, yellow for cancer and a white stripe to separate the two. Donal's words, *I have climbed God's Mountain and am at the top looking down*, are printed on the back, with his signature across the front. I have to contain my emotions as we leave Tralee, waved off by well-wishers, and head for Killarney. I have a group to lead to Moll's Gap and a tough road that needs my attention.

On a clear day, the view is magnificent along the pass to Moll's Gap. The road rises and falls, twists past glinting waterfalls and scattered boulders. Clouds float lightly across the mountain peaks when the weather is fine, but on the day we cycle the CrossDonalsMountain challenge, they lie heavily over the craggy slopes of the Macgillycuddy's Reeks and it's difficult to see beyond the grey haze. In one way, that helps, as I can't see how far the others have stretched ahead ... or the distance I still have to travel. Donal's bike, which I'm riding, is yellow as a canary but even its brightness is muted in this shrouded landscape.

Occasionally, as the mist momentarily clears, I see his words on the back of the cyclist in front and that urges me onwards. As I climb the steep inclines and relax on the downward slopes, I think of him, breathing in the same clear mountain air the previous year, his young heart beating fast with the energy of life.

I feel contented when we reach Moll's Gap. 'There you go, Donal,' I tell him. 'I've kept my promise. I've done it.' We've raised €7,500 for CROSS. Mick Galwey recalls his meeting with Donal at Moll's Gap the previous year and how he, along with some of the other legends, cycled part of the journey with him. They thought he was incredibly brave to undertake the stage so soon after recovering from surgery. Donal and Mick led the group back into Tralee, which for Mick, who is a Kerry man, was a great moment. Little did anyone realise then that twelve months later, Donal wouldn't be here to join us.

I intend continuing on from Moll's Gap with the legends and ending my cycle in Bantry. I'm saddle-sore by now and Donal's stainless steel bike is on the heavy side. For the next stage, I'll use my own lighter-framed bike. We set off at a fast pace, spurred on by thoughts of a hearty lunch. We have 100 kilometres to cover but the mist has turned to rain and it pours for the entire trip. This has become an endurance test. Is my son, mischievous as ever, punishing me for not using his bike?

Going up the Caha Pass, the real cyclists take off and the rest of us trail wetly in their wake. I hope for a rest-break at the top, but no such luck. They're determined to make Bantry for lunch. By the time we arrive in Glengarriff, I've reached my previous limit of 100 kilometres. Now, every extra kilometre is hell. I don't know if I can make it but I have Donal on my shoulder, goading me on. I reach Ballylickey and with only five kilometres to go, I ease back on the gears and cycle the home stretch. It has been a tough, gruelling cycle but I psyched myself onwards by remembering how my son cycled to the limit of his endurance with his prosthetic knee and severely depleted lung power. Somehow, as for many others who undertook the trip, my journey seems easy in comparison.

Chapter Fifty-Eight

There's hardly time to draw breath, before Elma and I are on the road to Dublin the following day for the People of the Year Awards. I'm aching from the cycle and take full advantage of the jacuzzi in the hotel. The People of the Year Awards recognises those who have made a real difference to people's lives over the year. The air of celebration is mixed with a sombre awareness that some of these awards are posthumous. We are deeply moved when Caroline Donohoe accepts a posthumous award that acknowledges the bravery and fearlessness of her husband, Detective Garda Adrian Donohoe, in carrying out his duty. We remember his callous shooting and the shock waves that rippled across the country when the news broke. Another brave recipient is Fiona Doyle, who is rewarded for her courage and determination to fight for her own rights and the rights of survivors of abuse. There's humour, too, as Brendan O'Carroll of the famed *Mrs Brown's Boys* takes to the stage to receive his award for his services to the Irish entertainment industry.

Then we hear Donal's name and rise to our feet to accept

the Joint Young Person of the Year Award, for his courage, strength, determination and his desire to show young people the true value and meaning of life. This is the first award we have received since his death, and it is important to remain composed. Brendan O'Connor presents it to us and speaks movingly about his encounter with Donal. 'I think that was meeting someone who was in a state of grace,' he says. 'Donal said he had put himself in God's hands by that stage and I think that's what it was. He radiated a certain peace and understanding.'

Gráinne Seoige, who is hosting the occasion, asks if we can believe the impact our son has had on Kerry and then the rest of the country. But it has gone much further even than these shores. I tell her that Donal's message has been translated into Cantonese, Portuguese and Swedish. My brother Kieran met an Indian businessman, who was on a trip to London for a business conference. He had heard of Donal and asked how a sixteen-year-old youth had acquired such wisdom. Pupils in a school in Australia have given him a posthumous student award. Word seems to be spreading almost by osmosis ... or, more probably, by the power of social media. Elma repeats Donal's message to young people. Live the life our son could not live.

The following day we fly to New York. We've been invited by Crumlin Hospital to speak at the Broken Arrow Golf Club for their annual US fundraiser. As we embark on the flight, I wonder when our lives will slow down, but this seems to be our new normality. We speak to the assembled guests, many of them Irish and Irish-American, and receive a courteous reception. It doesn't seem to matter where we speak – in schools, community centres, churches – the reaction is always the same. Silence, followed by questions and an eagerness to pass on Donal's story. On this occasion the annual golf tournament will raise $100,000.

The Irish Rugby Football Union approach us to ask if we can organise an event that will help spread Donal's message to the young people in the branches and grass roots of the organisation. I remember the bed-push walk Donal and I had planned in such detail. He was fighting his second battle with lung cancer when it should have happened and, afterwards, we ran out of time. So there it is, a well thought-out fundraising strategy that can be undertaken in his memory.

I approach the committee of Tralee RFC with the idea of organising the walk, but without the bed. The club already uses the #Livelife logo on the main panel of their jersey and they are enthusiastic about supporting the idea. This will be a fundraising walk for Crumlin Hospital, #Livelife and Tralee RFC charities. The original idea was to connect with rugby clubs along the chosen route and I follow this plan. Each of the clubs I approach is eager to be involved. They plan to organise matches and other activities for the young walkers when we stop off at our different destinations. I approach the two schools in Tralee that the majority of our rugby players attend: CBS The Green and Mercy Mounthawk, the co-educational secondary school. I focus on the transition-year students and they, like everyone else, are delighted to be included. The IRFU and Munster Rugby want to be active participants in advertising and promoting the event, which will take place on 2 February 2014, when Ireland play Scotland in the first round of the Six Nations Championship in the Aviva Stadium. From there we will make our way in stages from Dublin to Limerick, and end up in Thomond Park.

The year draws on. We accept more awards in Donal's memory. The Irish charity Outreach Moldova – which raises funds for abandoned/orphaned children, children with special needs and children with terminal illnesses in the Republic of Moldova – presents us with the Spirit of Humanity Award. This is in recognition of the awareness Donal raised on paediatric illnesses and palliative care. For once, the focus is on the journey he took with his cancer, rather than his 'anti-suicide' message. I think that would have pleased him.

Donal posthumously receives the Hugh O'Flaherty Memorial Award that honours the Kerry-born priest Monsignor Hugh O'Flaherty, who helped save over 6,500 people from death at the hands of the Nazis. The chairperson of the Memorial Committee, Jerry O'Grady, says that Donal was the obvious choice for this year's award. 'We had so many very worthy recipients this year but as a committee, we believe that this year belongs to Donal,' he says. 'The selflessness he displayed, reaching out to people in need, deserves to be recognised. Just like the Monsignor, Donal, through his actions, has saved lives and will continue to do so.'

As if to reinforce these words, Terence Casey, the South Kerry Coroner, goes public again, and states that Donal's appeal to young people has considerably reduced suicide rates in Kerry.

He usually deals with eighteen such deaths in a year, between one and two a month on average. Since Donal spoke out, no cases of death by suicide have come before the Coroner's Court from March to August 2013. This is a great change, he declares, and one he hopes will continue.

Chapter Fifty-Nine

Christmas comes. A very different one this year. The fun and laughter of last year's Christmas Eve party haunts us. The thought of that empty room upstairs is unendurable. We know friends and family will call, their support never fails us, but we need something different for this first Christmas without Donal. We decide to spend it in Rome and celebrate Midnight Mass on Christmas Eve in St Peter's. Earlier in July, at the ordination of Raymond Browne, the Bishop of Kerry, we met the Papal Nuncio to Ireland, Archbishop Charles Brown. Knowing how difficult this first Christmas would be for us without Donal, he helped us acquire tickets to attend this ceremonial occasion. It is a simple solution and will allow us to express our very mixed emotions in an atmosphere that is both spiritual and celebratory.

Outside St Peter's Basilica we wait to be admitted. The queue is long and stretches back at least a kilometre. Here, we are part of an anonymous crowd, away from the spotlight, able to celebrate our memories of Donal in our own personal way. We're finally ushered into the basilica where, to our surprise, we are led up the centre aisle and seated about ten rows back from the altar. We have a perfect view of the entire ceremony and settle into the solemnity of the occasion. Music soars above us in magnificent waves as the procession of priests moves towards the altar.

We're moved by the simplicity of this new pope. The ritual by which every priest in the procession kisses the altar has been changed, and only Pope Francis with his two concelebrants performs this act of veneration. I have a knowledge of Italian, gained from my time in Rome, so I can understand him when he delivers his homily. Elma, who has no Italian, asks for an interpretation on a few occasions but, in general, his language is so simple that she is able to follow the substance of what he is saying. His words resonate with meaning and I hold back tears when he says, 'If our hearts are closed, if we're dominated by pride and deceit and the constant pursuit of self-interest, then darkness falls within and around us.' I think of Donal, and how he never allowed darkness to fall around him. Yes, he'd been angry and inconsolable at times during his illness but he'd battled those emotions as fiercely as he battled his cancer. The singing is both gentle and magnificent by turn. The choir swells in harmony or dominates the hushed atmosphere with a single, melodious voice. The ceremony lasts for two-and-a-half hours but the time seems to fly. In these splendid surroundings, in the midst of the glorious singing, the pomp and ancient rituals, Pope Francis celebrates his first Christmas Mass as Christ's Vicar on Earth. Like us, he too is facing into a new future. One that he did not choose for himself. But, having been chosen, he is walking a different path.

We return home to Kerry, renewed and rested. On the first day of the New Year we have a gathering in our house to watch a documentary of Donal's life. It has been filmed posthumously and will feature videos made by his friends, as well as clips from *The Saturday Night Show*. Friends, relations and his rugby heroes speak about him. We took no part in the editing, even though we were offered that option. During the filming we were interviewed about Donal and those final moments we shared with him. It was an emotional retelling and we hoped our grief would not be exploited. Our fears were put to rest when we watched a preview but now, surrounded by others, we hope we can watch it without breaking down.

The mood of the documentary is uplifting. The viewers see the positive, energetic Donal, enjoying his life to the full. A few weeks before his death, he was clowning around with his friends as they made a video of themselves doing a frenzied take-off of Justin Bieber. It's impossible not to laugh as we watch him having fun, and cry an instant later. He's so alive, so animated. There are tears and laughter as the documentary draws to a close. His friends have spoken eloquently and movingly, as has Jema, and the other young people who were interviewed. They did him proud, and themselves too. One of them joked that Donal used to say he'd make them famous one day, and now it is happening.

'Donal Walsh: His Story' is watched in over 230,000 households and seen by more than half a million viewers. The following day the RTÉ Player crashes because of the demand to view it on RTÉ Playback. RTÉ decide to show the programme once more at prime time the following Saturday evening. It will run in competition against *The Saturday Night Show*. How Donal would appreciate that irony!

But all this publicity is causing us to lose our identities. We are becoming known as Donal Walsh's parents, uncles, aunts, grandmother. My own mother, a woman with strong opinions and an equally strong sense of humour, rings me one day to discuss this identity crisis.

'I married Donal Walsh in 1953 and became Mrs Donal Walsh,' she says. 'He died in 1990 and I became Donal Walsh's widow. Recently, I attended a funeral in Thurles and was introduced four times by the parish priest as Donal Walsh's granny. After eighty years, don't you think it's time I had my own identity?'

She's amused rather than upset, and, in truth, none of us mind. I've become used to being called 'Donal', and wave aside apologies when people, realising their mistake, become embarrassed. I live with the title of 'Donal's dad' and Elma is 'Donal's mom'. It's just another way of keeping his memory alive.

Chapter Sixty

It's February 2014, one of the wettest in Ireland since records began. Storms lash the coastline, shattering jetties, boats and barricades. Boulders are flung into the air, trees fall like ninepins, distressed people wade miserably through floods. What is Donal doing up there? Doesn't he know it's time for the Donal Walsh #Livelife charity walk? We joke as the day for departure draws nearer, but it is a serious situation. Forty-six transition-year students have signed up to journey from Dublin to Limerick, with stops along the way in Naas, Kildare, Portlaoise, Roscrea, Nenagh and the final, triumphant stop at Thomond Park Stadium six days later for the Munster v Cardiff Rabo Pro12 game.

We aim to cover twenty miles each day, walking and, where necessary, being bussed to the next destination where the students will collect for the various charities we've chosen. I've taken a week off work in order to travel with them and will be cycling most of the journey. Everything has been meticulously planned and the support has been amazing, especially among the students of Donal's school, who jumped at the opportunity to be involved.

'It's something they feel privileged to be part of,' says Ellen McGillicuddy, the transition-year coordinator. 'There's a very strong sense of solidarity and loyalty to Donal at the school, and they're honoured to be ambassadors for his foundation.'

More volunteers have come on stream and, much to my surprise, fifteen of them are female. This is not something I had anticipated, and more female supervisors are organised for the trip.

Before the departure date, Elma travels to Dublin for a press launch in Crumlin Hospital. Driving through the gates and entering these familiar corridors will always be a difficult and emotional experience. At various stages over those four years, this place became such a vital part of our lives. We felt profound hope and unspeakable despair within these walls, and we will never be able to enter without those conflicting memories bearing down on us. Elma's reason for being there is to attend the installation of a nineteen-metre-long piece of Irish rugby artwork.

Some weeks earlier I'd received a call from a representative of the Irish Rugby Football Union. He was looking for a venue to install an impressive painting of renowned rugby players running through a forest. The painting had been used as a promotion for the Irish international team during the autumn season and, now that it is no longer in use, Crumlin Hospital were delighted to accept it. The painting adds a bright splash of colour to the hospital. Some of the little children undergoing treatment for cancer pose for photos with the rugby players who have turned up to lend their support and promote the #Livelife walk. Rob Kearney, whom we met at the People of the Year Awards, has arrived, along with Mike McCarthy, Jack McGrath and team manager Mick Kearney. The children are enjoying the occasion and Elma holds her feelings tight when she sees their wide, brave smiles and colourful headwear. We know only too well the love with which their caps were chosen. With all our hearts, we wish these small angels a swift and full return to good health.

Elma does an interview about Donal and the #Livelife charity walk. This will be broadcast over the Aviva Stadium public address system on match day, along with big-screen advertising of the walk by the IRFU in the stadium. We have a page in their match-day programme and there will be media interviews and a number of other promotions. All we need now is the weather.

On the day before the walk, Tralee experiences the highest tide the town has seen for at least fifty-one years. For the first time our house is on the verge of flooding, as the canal breaks its banks, flows across the road and reaches the edge of the doorstep. Once again we joke to cover our unease. Are Noah and Donal having a scrum up there? We pin our desperate hopes on Donal winning and, thankfully, there's no need for an ark. The water retreats before it enters our house but the signs are ominous. If this weather continues, it will make the walk extremely difficult.

Thankfully, by the following morning the rain has stopped

and we assemble, as arranged, to begin our trip to Dublin. 6.30 a.m. is an early start and it's a group of very sleepy, tousled teenagers who board the bus. We stop off in Portlaoise for breakfast. By now most of the students are beginning to feel normal again. Conversations are breaking out, along with a general air of excitement and anticipation.

When we reach Dublin, we assemble at Wanderers RFC where we're greeted by the Club President, Niall Crowley and by Lionel Mahon, who has organised the club as our first stopover. We're preparing to depart for the Aviva Stadium when, to the students' surprise, Kevin Kelly from the Home to Rome Cycle arrives. Like our group, Kevin is also on a mission. In June 2014, he and thirty-one other cyclists will leave their homes in various counties throughout Ireland and cycle to Rome to raise funds for cancer and palliative care. The Home to Rome Cycle will be challenging and cover 2,000 kilometres. The young people listen attentively as Kevin tells them about the cycle and how they plan to promote Donal's message. Donal's writings have been translated into Latin, transcribed onto fabric and rolled in a leather binder. At various stages during the cycle, a rider will carry this scroll a certain distance before handing it over to the next rider. I think of an Olympic torch lighting the way to its final destination, and hope passionately that this message of positivity will shine a light for some young person struggling with problems that seem insurmountable. When the cyclists reach Rome, Donal's message will be gifted to the city.

Kevin has brought along the scroll for the young walkers.

They too will carry these words with them as they walk towards their destination. Donal would be in his element if he were here, loving the atmosphere, the camaraderie, the hardiness of the adventure – yet it is his absence that has created this sense of solidarity, this determination to walk the dream we once planned together. It has a new shape now. Yes, we will raise funds for our charities but the driving force behind our footsteps will be Donal's message to life live fully and trust in the brightness of a new day.

We head for the Aviva Stadium and park our #Livelife bus in a prominent position. We've established six points of collection and the young people have no difficulty attracting the attention of the supporters as they pour into the stadium.

Donal was with me the last time I was here. I remember his excitement and, then, his despondency when England won. I remember shielding him from injury as he bounded his way out, hoping he would not notice my efforts to protect him. The grief I now feel is a measure of the joy he brought into my life in his short sixteen years.

Our walk has attracted a lot of media attention. There are interviews to be done, photos to be taken. I'm becoming increasingly anxious as the time draws nearer to kick-off. I'm always intolerant of stragglers, especially those who arrive late for the Presidential Salute. It's one of my hobby horses and I've been known to sound off on the subject on more than one occasion. But this time, the shoe is on the other foot and I end up being practically the last person to enter the stadium as the game begins. Under normal circumstances that would be easy to do without attracting attention, but not when I've been invited to sit in the VIP box with President Higgins and other dignitaries. And so I slide in late and apologetically to watch Ireland score a dominant victory over Scotland. The #Livelife advertising within the stadium runs throughout the match and the after-game collection is incredible. In total over €6,000 is raised in the space of three hours. We return to Wanderers where food is waiting for the hungry collectors, who finally have time to watch the match on the big screen. By 1 a.m., even the most determined party person is in bed, the boys downstairs, the girls upstairs – an arrangement that will be repeated each night of the trip.

We rise early on Monday and head the short distance to St Michael's School where we enjoy a hearty breakfast and are welcomed by Tim Kelleher, the principal. This is the first of fourteen schools I will visit during the week. When the transition-year students are assembled, I talk to them about Donal. I've become used to giving this presentation, as has Elma. Wherever we go, we're treated with respect by young students, who listen with interest to our story. They can relate to Donal, to the games he played, the music he enjoyed, the house parties he gave, his reaction to being on *The Saturday Night Show*, and, invariably, they want to hear about his illness. How he coped, when there was no hope left. We tell them about his fight, his desire to live every moment that was left to him. Two days in bed when he was no longer able to fight the ravages of his disease – that was all he allowed himself. But that silence greets us, no matter what the age of our audience or where we are speaking. Older people are deeply moved by our loss but I know that when they listen to us, they are linking our experiences into their own personal tragedies. Grief is a raw wound that is easily exposed. The more we talk to people, the more letters we read, the more determined we are to fight against this tide of youth suicide.

The rain has returned and the walkers face their first challenge as they head cheerfully and with great determination towards Crumlin Hospital. I will meet them there later after I've spoken to the pupils of CBS Monkstown. Again, I have the complete attention of my young audience and when I'm finished, the pupils present me with a gift of their school hoodie.

There are many highlights during this trip, but one of the most emotional experiences is my visit that same day to Crumlin Medical Research Foundation. We are received in the room where Donal and I had lunch on that fateful afternoon when Dr Capra phoned and told me to prepare myself. The memory hits like a punch to my stomach as I enter the room. What keeps me motivated is the knowledge that what we are doing on this walk – and other fundraising events I will undertake in the future – is bigger than my grief. Nothing will ever be bigger than my loss but if spreading Donal's message saves one young person from taking that fatal step, then I will cope, somehow.

Michael Capra talks to the young people about Donal and his achievements. They are particularly moved when he tells them that there are also good outcomes from this devastating disease. One of them is Jonathan Myers. We met him and his family in the Ronald McDonald House when Donal first became ill. Jonathan had also been on the same journey and, at that time, was undergoing radium treatment in St Luke's hospital. He and Donal became friends and our families bonded in the maelstrom of our sons' illnesses. And here is Jonathan now, fully recovered, and one of our walkers. I feel a lump in my throat when I look at this healthy young man, and thank God that some stories have a happy ending.

In St Mary's College in Naas I speak to three different groups of girls, then meet up with my walkers, who have had a tough day, weather-wise. The public have been kind to them, however, and the collection boxes are heavy. That night we stay with Naas RFC, where dinner is prepared by the club members. Afterwards, they are brought into the KBowl Entertainment Centre in Naas where they have a highly entertaining match against the transition-year members of Naas RFC. This is followed by a disco back at the club. Somehow along the way, the heavy rain that day is becoming a forgotten discomfort.

The following morning the volunteer chefs are up bright and early to cook our breakfast before we hit the road. All my efforts to pay for the plentiful food we've eaten fall on deaf ears. Before we head off, Anthony Lawlor, the local TD and one of the morning chefs, wishes us success before he heads off on his constitutional duties.

Tuesday follows much the same routine, with a visit to Naas CBS and our collectors receiving a very generous response wherever they stop. The pupils are open and receptive to my talk, and ask many questions. This is a good response.

Sometimes, I'm afraid I'll choke up during one of these sessions but when the questions come thick and fast, it makes it easier to overcome such fears. Is this my therapy, I wonder, as I take my leave. But I know my journey is far from over.

My physical journey, however, moves on to a radio interview on KFM and a cycle to Newbridge College where the walkers have assembled. It's all going according to plan, even if the itinerary is a bit stretched at times. We head for Kildare. Unlike yesterday, this is a perfect spring day and the flat plains of The Curragh are ideal for cycling. The walkers are in good spirits, and the craic between them is mighty as we reach Kildare town. #Livelife banners have been erected in the school walls and groups of students are waiting for something to happen. I'm not sure what they're expecting, but I suspect it's not a fifty-one-year-old cyclist in Lycra. After the talk ends, I'm approached by one of the older students who introduces himself as Luke Burke and asks if I remember him. He was one of the players who joined my rugby squad in 2006, two years before Donal's illness struck. I recall him now, a strong and sturdy team player. I'd been disappointed when he moved from Tralee and it's good to talk to him about those days, when the only thing I had to worry about was whether or not we won the next game.

We stay overnight in Cill Dara RFC. The club is playing host to a college rugby cup game between St Andrew's and Celbridge. The victory goes to St Andrew's, and the rugby players among the walkers are delighted at the opportunity to see Leinster college rugby in action. On the field I'm approached by parents and students from both colleges, to offer condolences and express their gratitude for the awareness Donal brought to the discussion on youth suicide. We're asked if we would consider visiting a local town where there have been a cluster of suicides, including one that has deeply affected a particular school. The school is not on our itinerary and we are under serious time constraints, but how can we turn down such a specific request? Is this not why we are here, in this place, spreading the #Livelife message?

The following morning the weather is atrocious. Our walkers are willing but it would be inhumane to send them out in it. After a brief discussion amongst the organisers, we arrange for a bus to take us to the school. To open the proceedings I invite Danny Cournane, who is among our walkers, to do the Haka. Danny is one of the youngest members of the group. He's studying for his Junior Certificate examination in June, and, strictly speaking, this walk is for transition-year students. But Danny was determined to come with us and, now, he performs the Haka with the same intensity as he did so movingly at Donal's funeral. Needless to say, he has the students' undivided attention. We hold two sessions for the students from Third to Sixth year. The emotion in the room is powerful. These students understand what I'm talking about. They have experienced grief, loss and the guilt that trails in the wake of suicide. The school chaplain is extremely grateful to us for taking the time to include the school in our itinerary. To have done anything else is unthinkable and, given the circumstances, this will be remembered as one of the most important visits of our #Livelife walk.

After that stop-off, we continue on to Monasterevin and stop outside the SuperValu store. The SuperValu chain has, to all intents and purposes, become our unofficial sponsors. Wherever we stop along the route, if there is a SuperValu store, we are fed magnanimously. We're heading to Portlaoise and I still have a long cycle ahead of me. I'm being driven by Billy Keane to the spot where I'll begin my cycle. The day is once again winging away from us and I change into my Lycra in his car to save time. It's not easy to do and not a pretty sight in the rear-view mirror. I'm sure this is strictly against the Rules of the Road, and only hope that the passing motorists are keeping their eyes averted.

I arrive in Portlaoise and present myself at the school. I'm too breathless to wonder at the haste with which a class is assembled to hear me speak. The pupils look slightly bemused but, as always, there is a respectful silence while I begin my talk. I hear Billy's phone ringing. He leaves the room to take the call. Before the class can ask any questions, he hurries back and whispers urgently in my ear that we're in the wrong school.

At that point I'm hijacked by the gardaí and we're rushed across town in the back of a squad car towards the right school. All we can do is laugh. Needless to say, texts are flying between the walkers and the story is growing wings as it spreads. Donal would have loved it. His father in Portlaoise in the back of a squad car with sirens sounding and blue lights flashing. What a way to deliver his message!

And so we continue. The rain, when it falls, is a merciless

deluge interspersed with bursts of sunshine. We travel to Roscrea where we meet a retired rugby legend. Seamus Dennison has the enviable reputation of playing in that historic Munster match against the All Blacks. Thirty-six years ago his famous tackle against All Black superstar Stu Wilson set the tone for that most celebrated victory in Irish rugby history. Here he is, waiting to greet us when we arrive at Coláiste Phobal Ros Cré, where he is the popular history teacher. He's organised similar trips with young people in the past and knows that by a fourth day of sleeping on floors, everyone wants the luxury of a bed. And that is what they get. The walkers stay with various families in the town but before they can settle down to sleep, there is a soccer match to be played against the Coláiste Phobal Ros Cré school team. Once again Danny kicks off proceedings with the Haka, which is enjoyed by all, and in particular by Seamus, who tells the young people that he played against the All Blacks on two occasions – once in victory and, on the second occasion, in a draw when he played for Ireland.

Two of our walkers have to return to Tralee for football trials but, otherwise, we're still together and spirits are high. Tomorrow we'll arrive at Thomond Park, where volunteers will be on hand to fundraise. This will give our walkers a well-earned rest in the VIP box and an opportunity to watch the rugby match in real time. But first, we have two more stops to make, and both will be difficult for me.

After leaving Roscrea College after a memorial Mass for Donal in the school chapel – this school where Donal's great grand-uncle is remembered from the 1940s as both a priest and a veterinarian – we head for Moneygall and a brief stop in Obama country, where we are greeted by the President's eighth cousin, Henry Healy, known locally as Henry the Eighth! When people see what the trip is about, they compliment the young people on their efforts, then generously donate to the #Livelife fund.

In the town of Nenagh I speak in three schools and to a group of parents at Nenagh Ormond RFC, who are hosting our stopover. This is another first without Donal and a poignant reminder of our last visit three years previously. He was a survivor of cancer then, fighting his way back to full health. Fergal Healy of the rugby club had invited him to present the annual Crumlin Children's Hospital Cancer Trophy to the winning team. We'd had an enjoyable day, mingling with the teams and enjoying the atmosphere. That same atmosphere prevails today, as the young people enjoy each other's company. Youthful energy never changes and the memory of that happier, hopeful time reflects back at me in their bright faces. I hear it in their voices, the sudden outbursts of laughter, their optimism and confidence. I want it to always stay that way for them, but they are on their own journey. All I can do is promote my son's message and hope that if shadows cross their paths, they will remember him. The trophy has now been renamed the Donal Walsh #Livelife Trophy.

Our walk is drawing to a conclusion. On Saturday we arrive at Old Crescent RFC in Limerick for a #Livelife challenge game. The walkers are still going strong and excitement is high as the end draws near. Once again, I'm steeped in memories. This club has a special place in my heart. The youth squads have played with the Tralee squads once or twice a year from the time they were seven or eight years old. When they heard that Donal had osteosarcoma, they came to Tralee and John Hogan presented him with a signed, framed photograph of the four southern hemisphere rugby players challenging the All Blacks at the famous match in Thomond that Donal and I attended. This is my first time to enter the club without him and the memory of that thoughtful gesture, which meant so much to Donal, adds to the emotion of the occasion.

For me, this walk has been a pilgrimage. It will become an annual fundraising challenge but it will never have the same impact on me again. On four separate occasions – in the Aviva Stadium, in the Crumlin Foundation, in Nenagh Ormond and now, here in Old Crescent – in these places that have strong associations with Donal, I've stood without him for the first time and faced my memories. They will never leave me but, for now, I can lay them gently to one side and bring our walkers on the last leg of their journey.

It has been a pleasure and a privilege to be with these young transition-year students. For all of us, the #Livelife walk has been a momentous occasion. Everywhere we went, we were treated with the utmost kindness. Schools and rugby clubs willingly opened their doors to us. We were fed and watered and waved on our way. New friendships have been made and there has been much laughter. But, mostly, what these young people will remember is the kindness of communities, the eagerness of people to reach out and hold on to the message of positivity Donal left behind. I've talked so much about him every day to groups large and small – yet each time it feels as if I'm telling his story for the first time.

On we go to Thomond Park where Simon Zebo is wearing a #Livelife wristband as a tribute to Donal and to our plucky volunteers, who are greeted with an enthusiastic welcome when they march into the specially reserved VIP box. Munster are triumphant against the Cardiff Blues. The score: 54–13.

Chapter Sixty-One

Four years ago I could never have imagined standing up in front of 4,000 students at the launch of the 2014 Cycle Against Suicide. The previous year only thirty-eight young people attended. What was it in the collective Irish psyche that responded so openly and so instantly to Donal's words? If his story is stripped down to its most fundamental elements, it reads like this. A young boy gets cancer, fights it, and fights it again when it returns. After some local publicity, he appears for nineteen minutes on a national chat show to talk about dying and the value of life. A short time later, he dies. How did he create such a reaction? Become such an inspiration to young people? Illness matured him beyond his years, but he was still just a fun-loving sixteen-year-old youth, not long out of childhood.

Was it those five catastrophic years of recession that almost broke our spirit and, indeed, caused many people of all ages to take their own lives? Some of these stories have been well documented and are heartbreaking to hear. Since the collapse of the so-called Celtic Tiger, the news has been unrelentingly grim. The bank bailout, the Troika, the loss of our sovereignty, cutbacks, unemployment, emigration, company closures, the property collapse and the struggle to meet mortgage repayments on inflated loans. We've had political scandals and numerous stories of deplorable waste and greed. And in between those headlines, a young boy spoke and people listened.

He touched people by breaking a taboo, and spoke openly about death, the reality we never want to acknowledge. We skirt around its presence and hope it looks the other way, even though we know that death, in its many guises, waits for all of us. Donal knew its guise and he was not afraid to face it. He wanted a full life and when this was denied him, he asked others to appreciate the priceless gift of health. His words were simple but he understood the complexities behind them, and never underestimated the struggle that many young people experience through depression and harsh personal situations. Seek help, he said. Reach out. Don't give way to despair because you always have the option of tomorrow. You have what I desperately want. The hope of moving forward into a better day.

Adding his voice to this crucial debate on suicide has encouraged more awareness, more openness, more discussion among young people. Suicide statistics can no longer be shrouded in apathy. They are frightening to study. In the 2012 statistics, Ireland ranked fourth highest in the EU for deaths by suicide among young people between the ages of fifteen and twenty-four. The majority of these victims were male. Donal railed against such terrifying statistics and this issue is one we will continue to address through our #Livelife Foundation and various fundraising activities.

Donal's words may be misinterpreted, may be judged to be 'too simplistic', but that all adds publicity to this conversation. It draws attention to a problem that has reached catastrophic proportions and becomes more acute when there is a level of peer acceptance from those who see it almost as a 'right'. When life gets tough, there's a solution at hand, they believe. But the preciousness of life should never be undermined in this way. That is one of the reasons why people responded when our son spoke so movingly about his own struggle to live.

Elma and I, and Jema too, have become accustomed to the media glare. It's not always comfortable, and can sometimes be emotionally draining, to speak so openly about the son we lost. But the cameras don't bother us now. All we care about is the message and the future of our young people, who have so much living to do. We speak from the heart. We lost what was most precious to us and that gives our own words substance.

Elma is training hard for the Climb Donal's Mountain challenge, which will take place at the end of September. She has taken over Donal's personal Twitter account and regularly tweets about forthcoming charity and fundraising events. In the past she would have been reluctant to even stand in for a photograph but she now speaks in schools, churches, at mental wellbeing conferences and in localities where there have been a cluster of suicides.

At the National Newspapers of Ireland Awards, Brendan O'Connor asked what Donal would have done with his life if he had survived. He allowed the question to hang there for a few seconds, then said the time had come to stop asking it. Donal had achieved his potential at sixteen years of age, a potential that could take some of us four score years and more to reach.

Sometimes, especially on such occasions, it's difficult to recognise the son we knew and loved. He was always just our boy. 'A messer', as Elma called him. Harder on himself than anyone else, and always ready to blame himself when things didn't work out to his satisfaction, whether on the field of play or in school. When he wrote his 'Suicide Letter', it was carefully constructed and considered. He knew exactly what he wanted to say and the fact that he wanted it published after his death showed how little he sought publicity. He didn't see himself as having an influence on anyone. All that concerned him was that his message would have the maximum impact and save lives.

If cancer had not struck, he would have gone on to live a full, active life, unknown outside his close circle unless – and with his determination it would have been possible – he was chosen to play for his much-loved Munster team. A contented and happy life. That was all we ever wished for him. He was just an ordinary boy with ordinary problems, until he was dealt the hardest blow a young person has to endure. How he endured his illness and the courage with which he fought back is what made him, and others like him, extraordinary.

This commitment to #Livelife, and the publicity surrounding his death, has helped somewhat in filling the vacuum in our lives. And life does move on. Jema is still Jema – independent, free-spirited and with a supportive circle of friends who help her cope with the difficult days. She's building her own life, attending third-level education and enjoying her media studies course. When qualified, she would prefer to work behind the camera rather than in front of it. She knows front of camera can be difficult but she has coped with great dignity during her television appearances when she has spoken about her beloved brother. She is still closely aligned to the #Livelife foundation and the work we're carrying on in her brother's memory.

Friends who rallied around us in those crucial final weeks have returned to their normal routines. The lads, who walked every step of the way with Donal, still call but a little less frequently now, although they still participate in events involving his memory. His sporting heroes, who gave so generously of their time, came to say goodbye and pay their respects at his grave. They have busy, demanding careers and other causes to champion. We were gratified when we discovered that Ronan O'Gara, unbeknownst to us, had included #Livelife as one of his charities for his sell-out testimonial dinner in Cork.

On some occasions when I'm particularly tired, and I'm contacted by someone with a fundraising idea that I know I won't be able to refuse, I think, 'Donal, I wish you'd kept your mouth shut!' Then I laugh, knowing he's laughing at me, and ordering me up and out again to do his work for him. The same thought comes to me when I'm climbing a mountain or cycling up a hill. 'Why am I doing this?' I wonder. But, of course, I know the answer. He demands it. His belief that every life is important cannot be allowed to wither away.

We receive wonderful news at the end of February. The documentary, 'Donal Walsh: My Story' has been nominated for an IFTA (Irish Film and Television Award). We are touched by the nomination and aware, yet again, how, in spirit, our son is with us all the time.

We witness much sadness on our journey through life without him, but we also encounter tremendous optimism. Elma, in particular, has seen it among the young pupils in the schools she visits. They want to fundraise: run, cycle, bake, read, sashay down the catwalk, climb mountains. They are the future and they want it to be different. If they can achieve this – and we have no reason to believe otherwise – we'd like to think that our son played his own part in creating the awareness that life only comes our way once, and we must cherish it. It's too easy, in times of recession, to lose sight of the light at the end of the tunnel. To stop valuing ourselves, or to feel that we are of little consequence. That no one hears our story. But Donal saw that light. He knew it would soon be extinguished but he still found hope and value in the time left to him. We would like to think – no, we *believe* – that he has journeyed into a greater light. God's arms, he called it – and it is this thought that comforts us daily.

We will always be grateful that we had an opportunity to say goodbye to Donal. We know that this is not always the case for others, who have lost their loved ones suddenly and tragically through suicide. That is why we want to continue the conversation Donal started. We want to grow the awareness of how a decision, made in a few seconds, to end one's life can have such shattering effects for so many people in the aftermath. We hope that these heartbreaking statistics can be reduced and that young people will remember Donal. We want them to appreciate how much he struggled to spend every extra day with those he loved. And we want people to reach out and open that door. It will never be closed as long as young people keep talking.

Epilogue
Donal's Story

Some days I would wake up and I could easily appreciate the beauty of the world that I was leaving behind, although it does make me upset that I will never get to experience the feeling of living that I had on the bike or in the gym; or that I will never get to see my sister walk up the aisle next to the love of her life; or that I will never get to travel the world and see places like New Zealand, Asia or America; or that I won't get the chance to see my four best friends do as well in life as I know they will. But I have to remember that God is using me – whether He is using me as a symbol for people to appreciate life more, or whether His first two mountains weren't high enough for me, all I know is that I am walking with Him even though it is along His path.

I would like to take this chance to thank the people who asked not to be named but who have made a difference to the past few months for me and my family, whether they are other family members, businessmen or complete strangers. Thank you.

Acknowledgements

There are too many friends to acknowledge them individually for all the support that we have received over the five years of this journey, but if we leave someone out then we apologise. You all know what you did ... Family and friends, clubs and contacts, our employers Casey & Co. as well as the Gleneagle Hotel Group, especially Patrick & Eileen O'Donoghue, all who have taken us and www.Donalwalshlivelife.org under their wing and everyone who has supported us both in our grief and in this ongoing campaign. Special mention to Val from Tierney's who tried valiantly to retrieve the second half of the story when it disappeared from my laptop. Despite our best efforts, the *repairoso* spell didn't work.

Tralee RFC, Kerins O'Rahillys, his GAA club where he won an under-12 county medal, the IRFU and Munster Rugby. They have been behind us as a family since the onset of his cancer and have given us days that we could only dream of. Both his schools in Tralee, The Spa and CBS The Green, and other schools in the locality where his friends have attended are continuing to be part of our lives.

The staff of Tralee General (Cashel Ward), Crumlin, Cappagh, CUH and Marymount Hospice as well as the Palliative Care Unit from Tralee, especially Patricia Sheahan who cared for Donal on his final journey. At every point their care for him exceeded what was necessary. I do wish to thank everyone who had contact with him from the outset in his illness as there was never an issue with his care; you too, Peter!

To Brendan O'Connor, RTÉ, Independent News and Media and all the press who have broadcast or written about Donal – thank you for your kindness in dealing with us. You have proven that the story/issue is more important than the personalities. Most of these are now available to view or listen to on the www.Donalwalshlivelife.org site.

To June Considine for pulling this all together – yep it was my diaries and notes but I'm not the best writer in the world – and Ciara Doorley and Hachette Books Ireland for having the balls to ask if I have ever thought of doing this. Finally to Marianne Gunn O'Connor, the person who likes to say no, and Billy Keane for seeking her out for me! Ye all understand what I'm on about!

This is my story about Donal and his family. Friends have had input, but their story may come out in the future, and as my brother Seán says, 'On a journey like this each story may be different but it is from that person's perspective!'

To all who have been and are part of this ongoing journey ... Thank you & #Livelife!

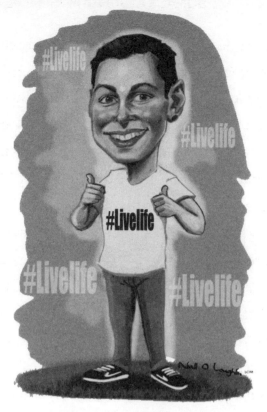

www.donalwalshlivelife.org
@DonalLiveLife

#livelife

Donations to the Donal Walsh Live Life Foundation will be used
to assist in continuing the conversation Donal started to prevent
teenage suicide. Thereafter, funds available will be utilised to
offer teenage-appropriate rooms in various care facilities.

By cheque to: The Donal Walsh #Livelife Foundation,
Hare Street, Blennerville, Tralee, County Kerry, Ireland

By bank transfer to: Permanent TSB,
Castle Street, Tralee, County Kerry, Ireland

Account name:
The Donal Walsh #Livelife Foundation
Account number: 21985820
Sort code: 99-07-11

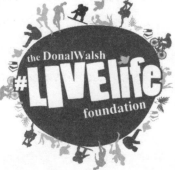